*Francis K. O. Yuen
Gregory J. Skibinski
John T. Pardeck
Editors*

# Family Health Social Work Practice
## *A Knowledge and Skills Casebook*

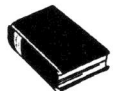

*Pre-publication
REVIEWS,
COMMENTARIES,
EVALUATIONS...*

"For almost a century, social work theoreticians and practitioners have been struggling to achieve the aspiration of a practice perspective that is family centered. *Family Health Social Work Practice* builds on the pioneering work of Mary Richmond, and is a valuable addition since it represents a marriage of both family and health. Yuen, Skibinski, and Pardeck differentiate the family health perspective from other approaches to practice. The book provides a clear articulation of the family health practice perspective and a rich array of case vignettes from several fields of practice, to enable the reader to understand its application to the requirements of everyday practice. The authors discuss family health policy as well as principles for organizing a family health agency.
Both students and professional practitioners will find the book of value since it distinguishes family health practice from specializations, generalists, and advanced generalists. The family health perspective describes a model of practice well suited to contemporary society with its ever-changing problem configurations."

**Roland G. Meinert, PhD**
*President, Missouri Association for Social Welfare*

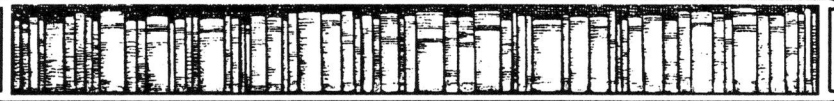

*More pre-publication
REVIEWS, COMMENTARIES, EVALUATIONS . . .*

"*Family Health Social Work Practice: A Knowledge and Skills Casebook* by Yuen, Skibinski, and Pardeck, arose from the need to provide social work education literature for the family health graduate curriculum at Southwest Missouri State University. The editors have made pioneering efforts to define the meaning of family health practice, to summarize family health research, and to provide a theory base for this emerging advanced social work curriculum. They have integrated family health with human behavior and the social environment, diversity and cultural competency, values and ethics, populations at risk, economic and social justice, policy and planning, and research and evaluation so that there are no questions as to how this specialty fits into the professional foundation social work curriculum.

The book provides ten case studies where family health practice is illustrated and applied in terms of assessment and intervention for students to make the connection between theory and practice. Case study areas are far-ranging: child maltreatment, domestic violence, mental health, child and family medicine, older adult populations, substance-abusing families, the spiritually diverse person, family services, the disabled, and family policy.

Program and practice model applications and summary principles of family health enhance this volume so that any social work program with an interest in health care and the family is provided with sold material for teaching."

**Doman Lum, PhD, ThD**
*Professor of Social Work,
California State University,
Sacramento*

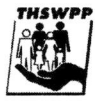

The Haworth Social Work Practice Press
An Imprint of The Haworth Press, Inc.
New York • London • Oxford

### NOTES FOR PROFESSIONAL LIBRARIANS AND LIBRARY USERS

This is an original book title published by The Haworth Social Work Practice Press, an imprint of The Haworth Press, Inc. Unless otherwise noted in specific chapters with attribution, materials in this book have not been previously published elsewhere in any format or language.

### CONSERVATION AND PRESERVATION NOTES

All books published by The Haworth Press, Inc. and its imprints are printed on certified pH neutral, acid free book grade paper. This paper meets the minimum requirements of American National Standard for Information Sciences-Permanence of Paper for Printed Material, ANSI Z39.48-1984.

# Family Health Social Work Practice
*A Knowledge and Skills Casebook*

# THE HAWORTH SOCIAL WORK PRACTICE PRESS
Social Work Practice
with Children and Families
John T. Pardeck, Senior Editor

*Family Health Social Work Practice: A Knowledge and Skills Casebook* edited by Francis K. O. Yuen, Gregory J. Skibinski, and John T. Pardeck

New, Recent, and Forthcoming Titles of Related Interest

*Principles of Social Work Practice; A Generic Practice Approach* by Molly R. Hancock

*Social Work Practice: A Systems Approach, Second Edition* by Benyamin Chetkow-Yanoov

*Social Work Practice in the Military* by James G. Daley

*Social Work in the Health Field: A Care Perspective* by Lois A. Fort Cowles

*Social Work Practice in Home Health Care* by Ruth Ann Goode

*Social Work: Seeking Relevancy in the Twenty-First Century* by Roland Meinert, John T. Pardeck, and Larry Kreuger

*Social Work Theory and Practice with the Terminally Ill, Second Edition* by Joan K. Parry

*Elements of the Helping Process: A Guide for Clinicians, Second Edition* by Raymond Fox

*Building on Women's Strengths: A Social Work Agenda for the Twenty-First Century, Second Edition* by K. Jean Peterson and Alice A. Lieberman

*Children's Rights: Policy and Practice* by John T. Pardeck

*The Use of Personal Narratives in the Helping Professions: A Teaching Casebook* by Jessica Heriot and Eileen Polinger

*Human Behavior in the Social Environment: Interweaving the Inner and Outer World* by Esther Urdang

*Diagnosis in Social Work: New Imperatives* by Francis J. Turner

# Family Health Social Work Practice
## *A Knowledge and Skills Casebook*

Francis K. O. Yuen
Gregory J. Skibinski
John T. Pardeck
Editors

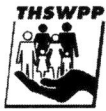

The Haworth Social Work Practice Press
An Imprint of The Haworth Press, Inc.
New York • London • Oxford

Published by

The Haworth Social Work Practice Press, an imprint of The Haworth Press, Inc., 10 Alice Street, Binghamton, NY 13904-1580.

© 2003 by The Haworth Press, Inc. All rights reserved. No part of this work may be reproduced or utilized in any form or by any means, electronic or mechanical, including photocopying, microfilm, and recording, or by any information storage and retrieval system, without permission in writing from the publisher. Printed in the United States of America.

PUBLISHER'S NOTE
Identities and circumstances of individuals discussed in this book have been changed to protect confidentiality.

Cover design by Marylouise E. Doyle.

**Library of Congress Cataloging-in-Publication Data**

Family health social work practice : a knowledge and skills casebook / Francis K. O. Yuen, Gregory J. Skibinski, John T. Pardeck, editors.
   p. cm.
   Includes bibliographical references and index.
   ISBN 0-7890-0717-7 (alk. paper)—ISBN 0-7890-1648-6 (soft)
   1. Family social work. 2. Core competencies. 3. Family—Health and hygiene. 4. Family—Mental health. 5. Medical social work. 6. Psychiatric social work. I. Yuen, Francis K. O. II. Skibinski, Gregory J. III. Pardeck, John T.

HV697 .F356 2003
362.1'0425—dc21

2002068754

To our spouses,
Cindy, Ann, and Jean,
and our children,
Amanda, Emily, Eric, Jon, and James

# CONTENTS

**About the Editors**     xiii

**Contributors**     xv

**Acknowledgments**     xvii

**SECTION I: ESSENCES OF THE FAMILY HEALTH APPROACH**

**Chapter 1. An Overview of Family Health Social Work Practice**     3
*John T. Pardeck*

| | |
|---|---|
| Family Health Research | 4 |
| Family Health and the Biomedical Model | 6 |
| Conceptualizing Family Health | 9 |
| Family Health and Systems Theory | 10 |
| Family Health and the Ecological Approach | 11 |
| Social Constructionism and Family Health | 12 |
| Generalist and Family Health Practice | 13 |
| Summary | 16 |

**Chapter 2. Critical Concerns for Family Health Practice**     19
*Francis K. O. Yuen*

| | |
|---|---|
| Human Behaviors and the Social Environment | 19 |
| Diversity and Cultural Competency | 22 |
| Values and Ethics | 24 |
| Populations at Risk: Economic and Social Justice | 26 |
| Policy and Planning | 28 |
| Research and Practice Evaluation | 32 |
| A Checklist for Family-Health–Centered Interventions | 33 |
| Generalist, Advanced Generalist, Specialized Concentrations, or Family Health Social Work | 35 |
| Future Directions | 37 |

**Chapter 3. Intervention Strategies of the Family Health Perspective**    **41**
    *Gregory J. Skibinski*

| | |
|---|---|
| Assessment and Diagnostic Impressions | 43 |
| Problem Sources and Manifestations | 46 |
| Intervention Skills to Eliminate Both Sources and Manifestations | 47 |
| Strategies to Evaluate Intervention | 49 |
| Example Case Study and Intervention Template | 51 |
| Conclusion | 53 |

## SECTION II: FAMILY HEALTH APPROACH IN PRACTICE

**Chapter 4. Child Maltreatment and Family Health Practice**    **57**
    *Gregory J. Skibinski*

| | |
|---|---|
| Assessment and Diagnostic Impression | 57 |
| Problem Sources and Manifestations | 58 |
| Activities to Eliminate Both Sources and Manifestations | 59 |
| Strategies to Evaluate Intervention | 62 |

**Chapter 5. Intervening with Domestic Violence Using the Family Health Perspective**    **65**
    *Joan C. McClennen*

| | |
|---|---|
| Introduction | 65 |
| Social Worker's Initial Interview with Rita | 66 |
| Assessment and Diagnostic Impressions | 68 |
| Identification of the Problem Source and Manifestations | 73 |
| Intervention Strategies and Skills to Eliminate Both the Sources and Manifestations of the Problems | 74 |
| Strategies to Evaluate Intervention | 76 |
| Conclusion | 77 |

**Chapter 6. Mental Health and Family Health Social Work Practice**    **81**
    *Catherine L. Hawkins*
    *Lisa Langston*

| | |
|---|---|
| Assessment and Diagnostic Impression | 81 |
| Source of the Problem and Manifestations | 85 |

| | |
|---|---|
| Intervention Strategies and Skills | 86 |
| Strategies to Evaluate Intervention | 88 |

## Chapter 7. Family Health Practice in a Medical Setting with an Infant and Her Family    91
*Melissa A. Hollis*
*Gregory J. Skibinski*

| | |
|---|---|
| Assessment and Diagnostic Impressions | 91 |
| Problem Sources and Manifestations | 96 |
| Intervention Strategies and Activities to Eliminate Both Sources and Manifestations | 96 |
| Strategies to Evaluate Intervention | 99 |
| Epilogue | 100 |

## Chapter 8. Family Health Practice with Older Adult Populations    101
*Christine A. Price*
*Francis K. O. Yuen*

| | |
|---|---|
| Introduction | 101 |
| Case Study: The Martinez Family | 104 |
| Assessment and Diagnostic Impressions | 106 |
| Problem Sources and Manifestations | 107 |
| Intervention Skills | 107 |
| Evaluation | 111 |

## Chapter 9. Navigating Family Health in Families with Alcohol Abuse    113
*James G. Daley*

| | |
|---|---|
| Introduction | 113 |
| Models of Family Recovery from Alcohol Abuse | 114 |
| Family Health Social Work Practice and Family Recovery Issues | 123 |
| Simulated Case Study | 125 |
| Future Directions for Family Health Social Work Practice with Families with Alcohol Abuse | 127 |

**Chapter 10. Family Health Practice with the Spiritually Diverse Person** — **131**
    *Francis K. O. Yuen*
    *Doman Lum*

| | |
|---|---:|
| Introduction | 131 |
| The Spiritually Diverse Person | 134 |
| Case Study: The Case of Annie | 137 |
| Assessment and Diagnostic Impressions | 140 |
| Problem Sources and Manifestations | 141 |
| Intervention Skills | 141 |
| Evaluation | 144 |

**Chapter 11. The Management of a Family Health and Family-Based Services Agency** — **147**
    *Francis K. O. Yuen*
    *John Gunther*

| | |
|---|---:|
| Family Health Agency Services | 147 |
| Building a Family Health Agency versus a Family Service Agency | 149 |
| Case Study | 153 |
| Assessment and Diagnostic Impressions | 155 |
| Source of the Problem and Manifestations | 156 |
| Intervention Strategies | 156 |
| Strategies to Evaluate Intervention | 159 |

**Chapter 12. Americans with Disabilities Act and Family Health** — **161**
    *John T. Pardeck*

| | |
|---|---:|
| Introduction | 161 |
| Discrimination and Disability | 162 |
| Harris Public Opinion Poll and the ADA | 164 |
| Case Study: Mary Ann and the Americans with Disabilities Act | 165 |
| Assessment Impressions | 168 |
| Problem Sources and Manifestations | 170 |
| Intervention Skills | 171 |
| Evaluation | 173 |

## Chapter 13. Family Policy and Family Health — 175
*John T. Pardeck*

| | |
|---|---|
| Problem Sources and Manifestations | 175 |
| Family Policy Supporting American Families | 177 |
| Evaluation | 180 |

## SECTION III: REFLECTION, SUMMARY, AND CONCLUSION

## Chapter 14. The Utilities of the Family Health Approach When Working in a Family Education and Support Program — 185
*Katie Ellsworth*

| | |
|---|---|
| Program Overview | 185 |
| Family Health Perspective | 186 |
| Comparison of the Family Health Perspective and the Family Education and Support Program | 186 |
| Family Health Practitioner Roles | 189 |
| Conclusion | 190 |

## Chapter 15. The Biopsychosocial Model of Pain Management — 193
*Mark J. Kellen*

| | |
|---|---|
| Introduction | 193 |
| Case #1 | 195 |
| Case #2 | 197 |
| Case #3 | 198 |
| Case #4 | 199 |
| Case #5 | 200 |
| Conclusion | 200 |

## Chapter 16. Family Health Social Work Practice: Summary, Problems, Focuses, Theories, and Intervention Skills — 203
*Francis K. O. Yuen*
*Gregory J. Skibinski*

| | |
|---|---|
| Definition of the Family | 203 |
| Dimensions of the Family | 204 |

Definition of Health     204
Definition of Family Health     205
Family Health Intervention Skills     205
Family Health Focuses, Theories, and Skills     206

**Chapter 17. Conclusions**     **213**
*John T. Pardeck*

**Index**     **219**

# ABOUT THE EDITORS

**Francis K. O. Yuen, DSW, ACSW,** is a professor in the Division of Social Work at California State University in Sacramento. Dr. Yuen is widely published in the areas of program planning, program evaluation, substance abuse, and services to refugees and immigrants. His interests in family health planning involve theoretical foundation, management and evaluation, community practice, and intervention skills.

**Gregory J. Skibinski, PhD, ACSW,** is a professor in the School of Social Work at Southwest Missouri State University in Springfield. Dr. Skibinski is the former director of the school's Master of Social Work program. He has published in the areas of child sexual abuse, social work practice, and program evaluation and his interests in family health include intervention strategies, child maltreatment, research, and health.

**John T. Pardeck, PhD, LCSW,** is a professor of social work in the School of Social Work at Southwest Missouri State University. Dr. Pardeck has published more than 100 articles in academic and professional journals. His most recent books include *Using Books in Clinical Social Work Practice: A Guide to Bibliotherapy* (The Haworth Press); *Reassessing Social Work Practice with Children;* and *Social Work Practice: An Ecological Approach.* Dr. Pardeck is a licensed clinical social worker and a member of the Academy of Certified Social Workers.

# CONTRIBUTORS

**James G. Daley, PhD, LCSW,** is associate professor for the Indiana University School of Social Work. His interests in family health practice include intervention skills, modeling, and substance abuse.

**Katie Ellsworth, MSW,** is a social worker at United Way of the Ozarks, Springfield, Missouri. Her interests in family health practice involve services to children and families.

**John Gunther, PhD,** is Director and Professor for the School of Social Work at Eastern Michigan University. His interests lie in management in family health practice.

**Catherine L. Hawkins, MSW, LCSW,** is Director of Field Education for the School of Social Work at Southwest Missouri State University, Springfield, Missouri. Previous publications include writings in the area of family health social work practice.

**Melissa A. Hollis, MSW,** is a social worker in the case management department at Cox Medical Center South, Springfield, Missouri. Her primary areas of responsibility are the neurology and oncology floors.

**Mark J. Kellen, MD,** is an anesthesiologist and a director for the Center for Pain Management, Rockford Health System in Rockford, Illinois. He is a diplomat of the American Board of Anesthesiology and has credentials from the American Academy of Pain Management. He is interested in the psychosocial model of health practice.

**Lisa Langston, MSW, LCSW,** is a clinical social worker at the Counseling and Testing Center at Southwest Missouri State University at Springfield and an adjunct faculty member of the School of Social Work at the University. Her areas of interest in family health focus on community mental health.

**Doman Lum, PhD, DTh,** is a professor for the Division of Social Work at California State University, Sacramento. He has numerous publications including several books on social work practice with diverse populations. He is also an ordained minister and has a strong background and interest in spirituality and human diversity.

**Joan C. McClennen, PhD,** is an associate professor for the School of Social Work at Southwest Missouri State University at Springfield. Her interests in family health concentrate in the area of family violence.

**Christine A. Price, PhD,** is the Aging Extension Specialist for Ohio State University Extension for Ohio State University, Columbus, Ohio. She is interested in women's retirement transitions and issues of aging families.

# Acknowledgments

Francis Yuen is thankful for the teaching, support, and understanding of his family. Greg Skibinski is thankful for the support of his family, friends, and colleagues, whose wisdom, assistance, and understanding helped make this book possible. John Pardeck thanks his supportive colleagues.

The editors appreciate the editorial assistance of Terry Brown, particularly on those last-minute turnarounds. We would also like to thank the chapter contributors for their dedication and insights into the family health practice. We are grateful for the support, patience, and expertise of the staff at The Haworth Press. Valuable critiques, encouragement, and insight from our students and clients have inspired us greatly in the development of this book.

# SECTION I:
# ESSENCES OF THE FAMILY HEALTH APPROACH

## Chapter 1

# An Overview of Family Health Social Work Practice

John T. Pardeck

Family health practice is an emerging practice paradigm in the field of social work. As a field of practice, family health has its seminal roots in the early works of Mary Richmond and other pioneers in the field of social work practice (Pardeck and Yuen, 1999). These early pioneers in the profession of social work realized the importance of the family system in the development and well-being of family members. Family health goes beyond, however, the more narrow policy and practice approaches presently found within social work because it stresses a holistic orientation to assessment and intervention with the family system. When practitioners conduct an assessment from the family health perspective they include physical, mental, emotional, social, economic, cultural, and spiritual dimensions of family life. Given this holistic approach to the family system, family health is defined as follows (Pardeck and Yuen, 1999):

> Family health is a state of holistic well-being of the family system. Family health is manifested by the development of, and continuous interaction among, the physical, mental, emotional, social, economic, cultural and spiritual dimensions of the family; all of these aspects result in the holistic well-being of the family and its members. (p. 1)

In a previous work, Pardeck and Yuen (1999) outlined the basic premises that guide family health social work practice as follows:

1. Family health social work practice is grounded in a biopsychosocial approach to assessment and intervention; it rejects the narrowness of the biomedical model as a practice approach.
2. Family health is based in a systems-ecological approach to practice because of the role that various systems play in the well-being of the family. These systems include the person, the community, and the larger social context, which includes the numerous social systems that impact family functioning.
3. Family health views the family as the most important system for promoting the growth and development of the person.
4. Family health social work practice requires close collaboration between social workers and other professionals. The complexity of problems facing families demands the help of many professionals; social workers must be able to work with these groups.

These premises form the grounding for family health social work practice. The research on family health suggests that these premises have empirical support.

## *FAMILY HEALTH RESEARCH*

Campbell (1986) conducted an in-depth review of the literature on family health, including more than 200 articles. Campbell reported that much of the research on family health is based on social epidemiological data (Pardeck, 2001). Campbell's review of the literature discovers evidence for the role of the family system in the development of asthma and diabetes in family members. He also finds evidence for an association between marital status and overall mortality rates and cardiovascular disease. Campbell discovers some support for the role of "psychosomatic families" in influencing physical illnesses. He finds a strong correlation in the literature between family support and compliance with medical regimes. Campbell reports that systems theory is the dominant paradigm in the family health research literature; much of this literature focuses on mental health problems. Last, Campbell reports a very large body of research literature focusing on the impact of the family system on alcohol and chemical dependency.

Ell and Northen's (1990) review of the family health literature supports many of Campbell's findings. Ell and Northen find that the family system as a result of the socialization process appears to shape family members' health practices and health services utilized. They reported that the family has an influence on the psychological health of family members in both the theoretical and empirical literature. Examples of the family's impact on psychological health include evidence suggesting that family loss may be etiologically implicated in the development of certain emotional problems. Family coping styles are associated with Type A behaviors in family members. The Ell and Northen review of the literature finds other studies for the association between family stress and the illness onset. This literature generally concludes that positive family supports enhanced family members' general well-being and the ability to cope constructively with stress (Pardeck, 2001).

Research by McDaniel, Hepworth, and Doherty (1992) summarizes the advances in the family health research into the early 1990s; these findings included the following:

1. The family plays a critical role in health practices of family members.
2. Illness stressors originating inside and outside the family system influence the physical and emotional health of family members.
3. Family beliefs about health and illness are important to successful treatment outcome.
4. Families go through predictable stages as they confront and deal with illness of family members.
5. The family's adaptation to illness has an important impact on family roles and the family system in general.

The work of Akamatsu and colleagues (1992) on the topic of family health offers additional analysis of the research and theory on the impact of the family in the promotion of health and illness. Their analysis suggests that the family plays a significant role in the physical and emotional functioning of individuals. Akamatsu et al. (1992) conclude that within the helping professions, particularly in the discipline of psychology, the role of the family in promoting health in individuals has emerged as a field of practice identified as family health.

A content analysis study by Thompson and Pardeck (2000) reports many articles on family health-related topics in the social work literature. Even though the term *family health* is new to the profession of social work, their review of the social work literature found numerous articles on topics related to family health. Their research employed the definition for family health presented earlier in this chapter. This definition includes the following: the physical, mental, emotional, social, economic, cultural, and spiritual dimensions of family health. Thompson and Pardeck's exploration of these dimensions in the social work literature reports that the family health dimension offering the greatest number of articles was the mental dimension of family health. The social and spiritual dimensions offer the fewest articles. Table 1.1 reports the top six journals in the field of social work and the number of published articles from 1977 to 1999 on family health topics.

This chapter is grounded in the proposition that families influence individual health and illness and, conversely, families are affected by individual members' health status. The research and theoretical literature clearly support this orientation.

## *FAMILY HEALTH AND THE BIOMEDICAL MODEL*

The biomedical model has played a major role in the strategies used to deliver health and human services in the United States. This model argues that pathology in human beings has a biological or mo-

TABLE 1.1. Top Six Journals Publishing Articles on Family Health Topics

| Journal | Number of Articles |
|---|---|
| *American Journal of Orthopsychiatry* | 20 |
| *Families in Society* | 13 |
| *Social Work* | 11 |
| *Hospital and Community Psychiatry* | 10 |
| *Social Casework* | 9 |
| *Child Welfare* | 8 |

lecular basis. As a treatment approach, the biomedical model has been very successful at curing many diseases. Given this success, professionals in a number of fields have been greatly influenced by the biomedical model in the assessment and treatment of both physical and emotional problems (Pardeck and Yuen, 2001).

McDaniel, Hepworth, and Doherty (1992) have presented an in-depth analysis of the limitations of the biomedical model. Their analysis concludes that the goal of treatment by those using the biomedical model is to identify the physical basis of disease and to treat it. The psychosocial aspects of illness are largely disregarded by practitioners using the biomedical model. The biomedical model has the tradition of dividing the mind and body into separate parts; this division has its origins in dualism, a perspective formulated by Descartes (Pardeck and Yuen, 1999). The biomedical model gives limited attention to the role that social systems, such as the family, play in the development of illness; thus diagnosis and treatment are narrowly defined (Pardeck and Yuen, 2001).

An emerging body of research suggests that the psychosocial aspect of illness must be a part of the assessment and intervention process (Neuman, 1989). For example, Engel (1977) in his research illustrates the importance of psychosocial factors in assessing and treating physical and mental illness. Engel concludes that the biomedical model's interpretation of illness is narrowly defined and disregards the importance of psychosocial factors in assessing health and illness in people. Research by Krantz and Manuck (1985) concludes that the root cause of atherosclerosis and essential hypertension may be better explained by examining the behavioral stimuli triggered by factors such as stress. In fact, a new discipline called psychoneuroimmunology is emerging that pinpoints psychosocial stressors such as major life adjustments, job-related stress, and family difficulties as capable of producing immunological deficits which increase the opportunity for illness (Danielson, Hamel-Bissell, and Winstead-Fry, 1993). This new area of research concludes that illness, both physical and mental, should be seen not only in biological terms but also in psychosocial terms (Danielson, Hamel-Bissell, and Winstead-Fry, 1993). The field of psychoneuroimmunology helps to legitimize the theoretical basis to family health social work practice (Pardeck and Yuen, 2001).

Figure 1.1 presents the theoretical grounding for family health social work practice. Using emotional problems as an example, a social worker might view the cause of an emotional problem from an extreme biomedical model. The treatment would thus be focused on the biological basis of the problem. Social workers using an extreme psychosocial model would disregard the importance of the biological basis of an emotional problem and instead focus solely on its psychosocial causes. Other clinicians might split their assessment and treatment of an emotional problem into parts consisting of the three aspects of the biopsychosocial. Some practitioners, as suggested in Figure 1.1, may locate themselves at various points on the biopsychosocial continuum, thus resulting in an emphasis of one aspect of the continuum over others.

Family health social work practice is located at the apex of Figure 1.1. Using a holistic approach, family health social work practice fully integrates the biopsychosocial aspects of a presenting problem; thus, assessment and intervention have a more realistic chance of positive intervention outcome. Family health views the family as a dynamic system that helps to maintain health, offers support to family members, affects health decisions, and attaches meaning to illness. In summary, family members under a family health approach are viewed as affecting and affected by the family system. Assessment and inter-

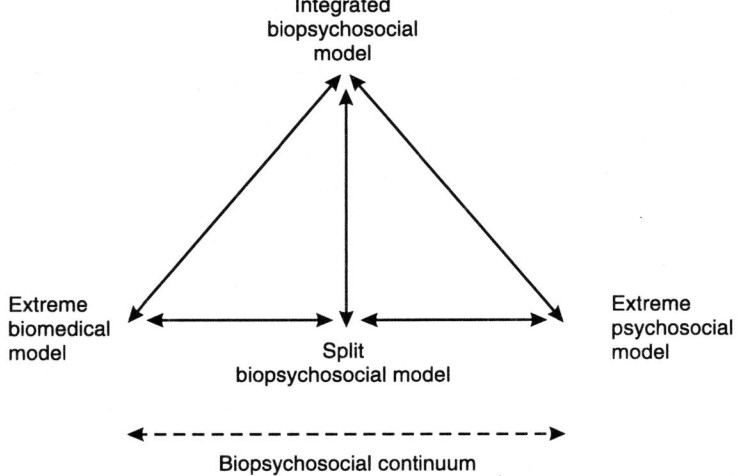

FIGURE 1.1. The Biopsychosocial Continuum for the Family Health Approach

vention from a family health perspective involves the biopsychosocial aspects of not only the individual but also the entire family system (Pardeck and Yuen, 2001).

## *CONCEPTUALIZING FAMILY HEALTH*

This book defines a family as a system of two or more interacting persons who are either related by ties of marriage, birth, or adoption, or who have chosen to commit themselves to each other in unity for the common purpose of promoting the physical, mental, emotional, social, economic, cultural, and spiritual growth and development of the unit and each of its members (Pardeck and Yuen, 1999).

This definition of family includes the nature, structure, and function of the family. It also establishes the boundaries for defining what is and is not a family. For example, one type of living arrangement that would not be considered a family is one in which a live-in girlfriend is boarding for the sake of economic necessity with a father and his children but is not committed to a unity for the common purposes outlined previously (Pardeck et al., 1998).

The following outlines each of the dimensions of nature, structure, and function (Pardeck et al., 1998).

The nature of a family is an important characteristic for defining the meaning of what is meant by the concept *family*. The family is the primary social system in society and is characterized by unconditional commitment to the total well-being of the family and its members. Individuals who share these traits, characteristics, or qualities can be classified as a family (Pardeck et al., 1998).

The structure of the family is the invisible set of functional demands that organizes the ways in which family members transact. A family operates through transactional processes. Repeated transactions establish patterns that underpin the functioning of the family system (Pardeck et al., 1998).

Family function comprises the activities necessary for the family to realize its common purpose which include the physical, mental, emotional, social, economic, cultural, and spiritual growth and development of family members. The functions of a family system are tied to the needs of the family as assessed by the family and larger society (Pardeck et al., 1998). A contemporary understanding of family functions suggests that particular states of the family, such as preparation for death, may be just as relevant as reproduction. Given this more modern view of the family, Pardeck and colleagues (1998) have identified the following functions of the family:

1. Physical care and economic security
2. Mental growth and development
3. Emotional nurturance
4. Socialization
5. Cultural transformation
6. Spiritual growth

These six functions contribute to the health and stability of society and families (Pardeck et al., 1998).

The term *health* in this book is defined as a state of holistic well-being. Health means being connected in a fulfilling way with the natural and human world (Pardeck et al., 1998). This definition for health is critical to understanding family health (Pardeck and Yuen, 1999).

## FAMILY HEALTH AND SYSTEMS THEORY

A system is comprised of individual parts; when change occurs in one part, all parts of the system are affected. Systems theory focuses on linkages and relationships that connect people (Pardeck, 1996).

Systems theory provides a paradigm that focuses on multiple levels of phenomena simultaneously and emphasizes transactional process. Systems theory helps social workers understand behavior in a social context and illustrates how systems impact individual and family functioning. Systems can be understood as open or closed; open systems are viewed as healthy systems, and closed systems are generally dysfunctional. This is a guiding principle of family health practice (Pardeck, 1996).

Systems theory as a theoretical approach moves away from a reductionistic view of human behavior by stressing wholeness as the key to understanding individual and family functioning. Component assumptions of systems theory include (Meinert, Pardeck, and Kreuger, 2000):

1. Wholeness suggests that change in one part of a system promotes changes throughout a system.
2. Feedback regulates a system through inputs.
3. Equifinality suggests that more than one way exists to achieve a final state of being.
4. Circular causality rejects the traditional scientific notion of cause and effect. Systems theory views linear thinking as being limited as a guide to understanding human behavior and family functioning.

Family health social work practice is guided by these assumptions, which means the family system is viewed from a holistic perspective throughout the assessment and intervention process.

## FAMILY HEALTH
## AND THE ECOLOGICAL APPROACH

Family health social work practice includes sensitivity to clients' worldviews and the ecological context in which clients function. An ecological approach is critical to a family health social work practice because it stresses the reciprocal, transactional, and holistic dynamics that exist between persons and their environment. Germain and Gitterman (1987) isolated the critical concepts of the ecological approach as follows: reciprocal causality/exchange, adaptedness, life stress, coping, niche, habitat, and relatedness. The ecological approach suggests that individuals and their family systems can be fully understood only in relation to the larger social ecology in which they function.

The ecological approach to intervention offers strategies for intervention at both the micro- and macrolevels. The ecological approach helps social workers better understand the impact of planning and policy activities on the family system. From a family health social work practice perspective and as noted earlier in this chapter, the family system is the most important system in the assessment and intervention process.

The ecological approach provides strategies that assist social workers in addressing problems and needs of families at various systemic levels. An ecological perspective offers strategies for helping social workers shift from a therapeutic role to planning and policy roles within a broad social context.

The ecological approach is clearly a holistic one that includes the individual, family, organizational setting, and community—all systems critical to assessment and intervention from a family health perspective. The following core assumptions guide the ecological approach (Meinert, Pardeck, and Kreuger, 2000):

1. Transactions are viewed as continuous, reciprocal exchanges that guide behavior.
2. Life stress can be seen as positive or negative within the person-environment relationship, which includes the family system.
3. Coping is seen as part of the problem-solving process and the management of dysfunctional behavior. The coping processes of individuals are largely shaped by their family systems.
4. Habitat is the social setting in which individuals and families reside.
5. Niche is the result of the individual's and family's accommodation to the social and physical environment.
6. Relatedness in one's environment supports attachments within the family system and the larger social ecology.

## *SOCIAL CONSTRUCTIONISM AND FAMILY HEALTH*

Systems theory and the ecological approach are critical theoretical underpinnings to family health social work practice. Both approaches, however, have limitations to which the family health social work practitioner needs to be sensitive. A major limitation for both theories is their tendency to deemphasize volition of the individual and the family system. Each approach also places entirely too much emphasis on the adaptation of clients, as well as the family system, to the social environment. A theory that can help the family health practitioner place systems theory and the ecological approach in their proper perspectives is social constructionism.

Social constructionism emphasizes that people have the ability to make sense of their personal experiences and to give meaning to reality. "Experiences of the objective and the subjective realms are selectively arranged on the basis of assumed themes, which organize, structure, and give meaningfulness to the person or family" (Kilpatrick and Holland, 1995, p. 25). A family health approach to social work practice stresses the importance of considering the family's view of social reality when doing assessment and intervention.

Social workers using the family health approach provide services to persons and their families at multiple levels. These services are designed to promote the holistic health of clients and their families and should facilitate the total well-being of individuals and their families. Families are active participants in the helping process when social work practice is conducted through a family health approach (Pardeck and Yuen, 1999).

## GENERALIST AND FAMILY HEALTH PRACTICE

Family health social work practice builds on generalist social work practice; however, family health has several unique differences from generalist practice. The following discussion compares and contrasts these approaches (Pardeck et al., 1998).

### Generalist Approaches

Generalist practice means the social worker can intervene at any systems level. Interventions based on the generalist perspective suggest that the social worker can bring about change in any system he or she employs. Numerous change strategies are available to the generalist social worker. These strategies can be used with a variety of systems including individuals, families, small groups, agencies, and communities (Pardeck et al., 1998).

The following definition by Kirst-Ashman and Hull (1997) provides an overview of generalist practice:

> Generalist practice is defined as application of an eclectic knowledge base, professional values, and a wide range of skills to target any system size for change within the context of three primary processes. First, generalist practice involves working effectively within an organizational structure and doing so under supervision. Second, it requires the assumption of a wide range of professional roles. Third, generalist practice involves

the application of critical thinking skills to the problem-solving process. (pp. 7-8)

This definition suggests that generalist practice is a blend of knowledge, values, and skills aimed at changing systems at the micro-, mezzo-, and macrolevels (Pardeck et al., 1998). A problem, however, of generalist practice is a lack of boundaries defining what is or is not generalist social work practice (Pardeck et al., 1998).

## *Advanced Generalist*

An educational "continuum" has been devised for defining the differences between generalist and advanced generalist practice. Advanced generalist practice is viewed as a specialty in graduate social work education; it is the grounding practice orientation for all accredited Council on Social Work Education (CSWE) undergraduate programs. Generalist practice at both the undergraduate and graduate levels includes the following roles: broker, advocate, evaluator, outreach worker, teacher, behavior change agent, consultant, caregiver, data manager, administrator, enabler, mediator, and community planner. What contrasts the two levels of generalist practice is that advanced generalist practice is defined less by the unique roles performed by masters of social work (MSWs) than by the expectations of greater depth and breadth of role performance at the independent practice level (Pardeck et al., 1998). Advanced generalist practice is seen as using generalist principles in a more independent, complex practice setting (Pardeck et al., 1998).

Advanced generalist practice is growing in popularity but is nebulously defined as an extra dose of generalist exposure. The boundary between where generalist stops and advanced generalist begins is not clear. Technically, the MSW graduate has the same skills as the undergraduate social work graduate; however, the MSW graduate has more exposure to how the generalist model can be used in more complex settings (Pardeck et al., 1998).

## *Family Health Social Work Practice*

Family health practice, from an educational standpoint, builds on the generalist framework with an in-depth understanding of family health. Family health social work practice uses a multimethod, multilevel, problem-oriented philosophy that is consistent with generalist practice. Family health social work practice is based on generalist practice; however, it offers a more complex understanding of the family as the focal point of assessment and intervention (Pardeck et al., 1998).

## *Advanced Generalist and Family Health Practice*

Advanced generalist practice builds on the multimethods, multilevels of generalist practice; these levels allow the social worker to intervene in more complex practice situations and to exercise independence and leadership at the micro-, mezzo-, and macrolevels (Pardeck et al., 1998).

Family health practice is grounded in generalist practice; however, the difference between generalist and family health practice is the centrality of the family system to family health practice. Expertise in family health social work practice adds an in-depth awareness and understanding of the family system that goes beyond the generalist approach. This orientation defines one's practice at all levels of assessment and intervention (Pardeck et al., 1998).

Generalist social workers have knowledge and skills that can be used at multilevels. Advanced generalists use this array of knowledge and skills at advanced levels in the areas of assessment and intervention. In contrast, family health social work practice stresses skills and competencies in working with families from a family health focus. Family health social work practice stresses knowledge based on the extensive literature on family health. Family health practice can be used in a number of practice settings including traditional health care as well as those focusing on mental health or children and family services.

Family health social work practice includes knowledge and skills for working with the physical aspects of health as well as the psychosocial components. Family health social work practice is grounded in the notion that the family plays a vital role in the physical and psychosocial well-being of family members. Family health social work practice uses assessment and intervention strategies at the micro-, mezzo-, and macrolevels. Table 1.2 offers the comparison of advanced generalist and family health practice (Pardeck et al., 1998).

TABLE 1.2. Comparison of Advanced Generalist and Family Health Practice

| Advanced Generalist | Family Health |
| --- | --- |
| Complex assessment skills | Adds perspectives on health and family to assessment |
| Problem solving | Problem solving and promotion of holistic well-being |
| Independent practice | Independent practice and expertise in family and health interventions |
| Broker of more complex situations | Interactional and reflective practitioner as broker of family health practice |
| Advocacy skills in more complex situations | Advocacy skills on complex health and family issues |
| Evaluator skills in more complex situations | Evaluator of health and family issues and practice |
| Expectation of managing skills in agency | Expertise in management of service systems serving health and family issues |
| Social justice view | Social justice view |
| In-depth awareness of family issues | Highly developed knowledge on family health issues |
| Policy analysis in complex situations | Policy analysis and practice in family health context |

*Source:* Adapted from Pardeck et al. (1998). Social work assessment and intervention through family health practice. *Family Therapy, 25*(1), 35.

## *SUMMARY*

This chapter describes family health social work practice as an invaluable perspective for helping families. Whether working to stabilize a family or prompt change, the social worker's target is the family system. Family health social work practice offers an in-depth understanding of family health grounded in generalist practice. This knowledge base allows a dynamic generalizability of skills needed for diverse clients and their families.

The family health practitioner has diverse skills and knowledge that allow him or her to work in many practice settings. The premises that guide family health practice are critical to how the social worker conducts assessment and intervention. Specifically, the practitioner uses a biopsychosocial orientation that is sensitive to the impact ecosystems have on the family system. Growth and development of individuals are largely shaped by the family system. The family health practitioner views practice intervention as a collaborative effort with other professionals. Last, the practitioner understands the self as "a part of" rather than "apart from" the helping process.

## REFERENCES

Akamatsu, T. J., Stephens, M. A., Hobfoll, S. E, and Crowther, J. H. (1992). *Family health psychology.* Washington, DC: Hemisphere.

Campbell, T. L. (1986). The family's impact on health: A critical review and annotated bibliography. *Family Systems Medicine, 4,* 135-328.

Danielson, C.B., Hamel-Bissell, B., and Winstead-Fry, P. (1993). *Families, health, and illness.* St. Louis, MO: Mosby.

Ell, K. and Northen, H. (1990). *Families and health care: Psychosocial practice.* New York: Aldine de Gruyter.

Engel, G. L. (1977). The need for a new medical model: A challenge for biomedicine. *Science, 196,* 129-136.

Germain, C. B. and Gitterman, A. (1987). Ecological perspective. In A. Minahan (Ed.), *Encyclopedia of social work,* Eighteenth edition (pp. 488-499). Silver Springs, MD: National Association of Social Workers.

Kilpatrick, A. and Holland, T. (1995). *Working with families.* Needham Heights, MA: Allyn & Bacon.

Kirst-Ashman, K. K. and Hull, G. H. (1997). *Generalist practice with organizations and communities.* Chicago: Nelson Hall.

Krantz, D. S. and Manuck, S. B. (1985). Measures of acute physiologic reactivity to behavioral stimuli: Assessment and critique. In A. M. Ostfield and E. E. Eaker (Eds.), *Studies of cardiovascular diseases* (pp. 10-16). United States Department of Health and Human Services, Publication no. 85-2270.

McDaniel, S. H., Hepworth, J. H., and Doherty, W. J. (1992). *Medical family therapy: A biopsychosocial approach to families with health problems.* New York: Basic Books.

Meinert, R., Pardeck, J. T., and Kreuger, L. (2000). *Social work: Seeking relevancy in the twenty-first century.* Binghamton, NY: The Haworth Press.

Neuman, B. (1989). *The Neuman systems model,* Second edition. Norwalk, CT: Appleton and Lange.

Pardeck, J. T. (1996). *Social work practice: An ecological approach.* Westport, CT: Auburn.

Pardeck, J. T. (2001). Clinical instruments for assessing and measuring family health. *Family Therapy, 27*(3), 179-189.

Pardeck, J. T. and Yuen, F. K. O. (Eds.) (1999). *Family health: A holistic approach to social work practice.* Westport, CT: Auburn.

Pardeck, J. T. and Yuen, F. K. O. (2001). Family health: An emerging paradigm for social workers. *Journal of Health and Social Policy, 13*(3), 59-74.

Pardeck, J. T., Yuen, F. K. O, Daley, J., and Hawkins, K. (1998). Social work assessment and intervention through family health practice. *Family Therapy, 25*(1), 25-39.

Thompson, R. and Pardeck, J. T. (2000). An exploration of the themes and content on family health in the social work literature. *Early Child Development and Care, 161,* 15-31.

# Chapter 2

# Critical Concerns for Family Health Practice

Francis K. O. Yuen

The goals of family health social work interventions are to restore, maintain, or achieve the holistic wellness of the individuals and the family. Practitioners competent in their family-health-grounded professional knowledge and intervention skills should also be sensitive to issues related to the social environment, human diversity, values and ethics, populations at risk, advocacy and social justice, political economy, and research and practice evaluation. This chapter discusses the relevance and importance of these concerns in relation to family health practice. It also presents a checklist which facilitates the inclusion of these concerns throughout the intervention process.

## *HUMAN BEHAVIORS AND THE SOCIAL ENVIRONMENT*

The family health approach is grounded in the understanding and intervention of the clients' ecosystems, for example, the person-in-environment and diversity considerations. "The theoretical orientations of the family health approach include the systems theory, ecological perspectives, social constructionist perspective, developmental theories, and other relevant family theories" (Yuen, 1999, p. 18). Figure 2.1 illustrates the settings and connections among the different components of the technology of a family health social work approach. The systems theory and ecological perspectives describe the context in which transactions among individuals, families, and their

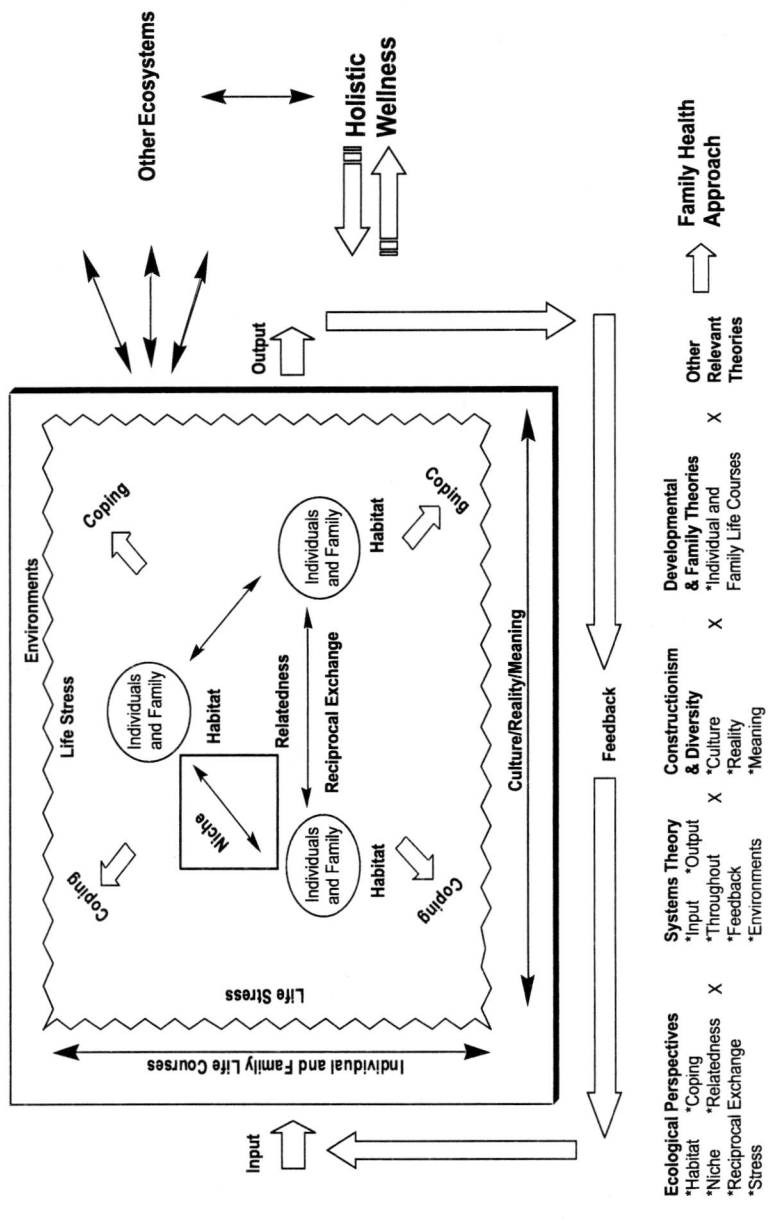

FIGURE 2.1. Theoretical Orientations for Family Health Approach

environments occur. "Social constructionist perspectives and developmental theories allow the subjective meaning and the reality of growth and change to be considered in the transactions" (Yuen, 1999, p. 18).

Ecologically, individuals and families as habitats occupy and develop their particular niches within their environment; their existence and reciprocal exchanges with others form the relatedness along with the life experience of rewards and growth as well as stress and difficulties. Individuals and families develop particular coping strategies, meaningful to their culture and reality, to deal with various life stresses throughout the different stages of individual and family life courses.

From a systems theory perspective, if individuals or families behave as open systems that have continuous input, output, and feedback, they continue to develop, and this may result in the attainment of the state of homeostasis or equilibrium. If the environments in which they reside exist as closed systems, they eventually become extinct. These environments also interact and network constantly with other ecosystems. Family health social work practitioners should develop the ability to understand the dynamics within and among these ecosystem networks to form the basis for designing proper interventions. These abilities may start with the exploration of the following sample questions:

- Who is involved, from the immediate to the extended environments? Who makes up the habitats?
- What kinds of niches do individuals or families occupy? How did these niches come about? How do the individuals or families perceive themselves and their niches in their environment? How do others perceive them?
- How have these niches positively and negatively affected the individuals or families in relation to other people and institutions in the environment?
- What kinds of stresses, both recent and chronic, have the individuals or families experienced?
- What types of coping strategies have the individuals or families been using? How successful are these strategies?
- What are the strengths of these individuals and families? How can these strengths be utilized, and what more is needed?

- What are the input, throughput, output, and feedback for the family, the individuals, and the presenting problems?
- What is the desirable homeostatic state according to the individuals or families as well as to others who are involved?
- What are the stages or extent of development for the individuals and the families? These may include stages in the family life cycle, physiological growth, and psychological and social development.

## *DIVERSITY AND CULTURAL COMPETENCY*

The family health social work approach includes culture and cultural diversity as integral parts of its theoretical and practice frameworks. Although different cultures have specific meanings and practice for the notions of health and family, the attainment of the well-being of the family and its members appears to be a common goal across cultures.

The United States is a multicultural society, and social work practitioners should take into consideration the existence of different cultural beliefs and practices. No "one size fits all" generic exists, nor does any all-purpose social work assessment and intervention approach apply to all cultures. Interventions have to be refined to fit the clients' cultural context. Clients' perceptions and meanings of events and issues, along with other personal, social, economic, and environmental factors, form the person-in-environment context for the formation and implementation of social work interventions. Diversity among people and cultures calls for social workers to formulate differential and culturally appropriate interventions in working with clients of different backgrounds.

In general usage, cultural awareness, cultural sensitivity, cultural diversity, cultural pluralism, and multiculturalism are mostly interchangeable terms. Practically and academically, each has specific connotations. The awareness of cultural diversity or human diversity suggests the acknowledgment of the existence of people of different cultures. People who accept culture diversity do not remain culturally apathetic and are well aware of different cultures. This cognitive understanding or acknowledgment may or may not transform into more or fewer intercultural interactions. Cultural awareness is merely the beginning of the recognition that "my culture is not the only one that is available." Such awareness does not, however, preclude attitudes that range from "mine is the best one and yours is useless" to "I like to learn, experience, and appreciate different cultures."

Starting at the level of cultural awareness, individuals of different backgrounds who are culturally aware interact in a manner that is sensitive to one another's culture. To a great extent, the popularity of intercultural or cross-cultural communication training in the past two decades in communities and the workplace has been the result of people trying to become more culturally sensitive. Often, these cultural sensitivity skills can be well performed behaviorally; they are, however, no guarantee of attitude changes. People may say or behave in the so-called right ways just to show their acceptance of diversity or to avoid the impression of being culturally ignorant. To some it is a politically correct thing to do; they may, in fact, have deep resentments toward all "diversity talk."

Cultural pluralism implies the recognition, the intention, and the practice of working with people of different backgrounds. It involves the advancement from cultural awareness to cultural sensitivity, and development of the ability to effectively interact cross-culturally. Cultural pluralism treats all cultures as equal and valid and asserts that all should be respected. Some have criticized the extreme forms of pluralism as "everything goes" and therefore lacking boundary and specificity to guide intercultural interaction as well as professional practice.

Multiculturalism not only recognizes differences and similarities among diverse cultures but also requires a framework of thinking that is inclusive and transcultural. This framework demands the ability to develop beyond cultural sensitivity to the level of cultural competency in interacting with people of various backgrounds. It requires one to think and act not only from the ethnically or culturally specific perspective but also from a multiple and collective perspective that allows one to conceive of common good and understanding among all people.

The idea of cultural diversity and the development of multiculturalism have generated many academic, social, and political discussions in the past decades. Although some have embraced the values of diversity and strive to become more competent in accepting and living with people of different backgrounds, some have questioned it as merely a movement of political correctness, which overrepresents the minority perspective.

Human diversity is an essential part of any family health social work practice. The different niches that individuals or families occupy in their ecosystems represent the basic diversity of the ecology. How each individual and family perceives its situation or stress and its choice of coping strategies is affected by cultural belief and practice. In family health, diversity comprises more than ethnic or cultural group difference; it also includes people of different sexual orientations, gender, physical or mental disability, and religious belief or practices of spirituality.

## *VALUES AND ETHICS*

Values refer to a set of preferences that people consider significant and important. Values are about "right" and "wrong." In daily language, this is expressed in the form of "should," for example, people should respect each other. Each individual, family, community, and society over time has developed, or at least claims to have developed, many core or basic values. These values form the basis and frame of reference for people to help them to make choices and to guide their behaviors.

Values are achieved through the development and use of knowledge. Knowledge is about facts. It concerns "true" or "false" and is expressed in the form of "being," for example, what is, was, or will be: "There are more female social workers than male social workers." Values set the parameter for knowledge and, in turn, knowledge helps to fulfill these values.

For example, social workers who prefer the residual idea of social welfare will likely be interested in acquiring knowledge and skills that help clients who have failed to fix their problems get back on their own feet. On the other hand, social workers who use the institutional concept of social welfare will likely be interested in learning knowledge and skills that promote social changes through policy and community organization. In many situations, however, the advancement of knowledge changes the existing values and the parameters of those values. Similarly, a change of values also brings about changes in the knowledge needed. Values and knowledge have a reciprocal relationship.

Values-guided knowledge often is used as the guideline for people's behaviors and actions. When practitioners in a profession organize the profession's values through a formal mechanism such as the professional society, and put them into action to serve as guidelines and standards for professional conduct and behaviors, these standards then become the profession's basic code of ethics. All established professions have developed a code of ethics to ensure quality and accountability to the clients and communities they serve.

The social work profession is based on a number of common values that, ironically, are not yet universally agreed upon by social workers. Often, social work values are discussed in general terms, or they are indicated throughout social work books and literature but seldom explicitly listed. The lack of a listing, however, does not indicate the absence of such values. Respect for human dignity, mutual responsibility among people, and belief in the possibility of change in people and systems are usually cited as the most basic social work values.

In past decades, through professional organizations such as the National Association of Social Workers (NASW) and the Council on Social Work Education (CSWE), the social work profession in the United States has developed a code of ethics that professional social workers are expected to adopt. Family health social work practices conform to the NASW Code of Ethics in the delivery of their services. However, additional cultural and ethical concerns exist that are of special significance to family health practice.

For example, a family health social worker who encourages individual growth, assertiveness, and achievement for a male teen immigrant from Mexico may find that he or she is unintentionally pushing the teen away from his family and culture. The youth is being empowered to become an achiever, while the parents become less and less in control of their children and family. The youth becomes the key person in the family because he is the family's cultural and social linkage to mainstream American society. Meanwhile the parents, who have been hardworking farm laborers, may become so-called undereducated and unsophisticated folks from the backward old country. These types of role reversal and selected growth do not take the family's holistic well-being into consideration. It is a child-centered, but not necessarily family-centered, practice. Interventions provided to this teen Mexican immigrant and his family are then concerns of clinical, ethical, and cultural competencies that need further holistic and reflective considerations.

Family health social work practitioners should expect to encounter ethical dilemmas in their daily professional practice. These practitioners need to be sensitive to the ethical implications of their interventions on the family and its members. How will one handle confidentiality, duty to warn, informed consent, cooperation with colleagues and other professionals, self-determination, and many other ethical issues in delivering family health practice? Ongoing education in the areas of practice theories, skills, and ethical decision making is essential in maintaining and increasing one's competency. Such professional education and development can be achieved through workshops and formal education in addition to growth through practice experience and professional supervisions.

## *POPULATIONS AT RISK: ECONOMIC AND SOCIAL JUSTICE*

Abbott (1919) reflected on Mary Richmond's orientation and reported, "the good social worker, says Miss Richmond, doesn't go on helping people out of a ditch. Pretty soon she begins to find out what ought to be done to get rid of the ditch" (p. 13).

Family health social work practice places strong emphasis on working with populations that are at risk and affected by discrimination and oppression. Ethnic minorities, women, people with disabilities, and gays and lesbians are among the many groups that are at highest risk. DuBois and Miley define social justice as "the social condition that enables all members of a society to share equally in the rights and opportunities afforded by society and in the responsibilities and obligations incurred by their membership in society" (1996, pp. 56-57). Often particular individuals or groups are denied opportunities to participate. According to DuBois and Miley, "full participation in society means that individuals have access to the social benefits of society in order to realize their own life aspirations, and, in turn, that they contribute to social well-being" (p. 57).

*Stereotype, prejudice, discrimination,* and *oppression* are terms often used in the social work literature. As a profession, social work commits to social justice and values diversity. Part of the preparation for becoming a professional social worker is to learn to overcome discrimination and to promote social justice. The term *stereotype* is the oversimplification and overgeneralization of a particular group of individuals based on few characteristics. It is an ill-informed knowledge that may include both positive and negative attributes of the group. For example, a stereotype exists that Asian-American students do well in school, excel at math, but do not have the capacity to be good managers. *Prejudice* is a negative attitude that is based on stereotypical knowledge. This attitude is a belief that may or may not turn into action. However, when one acts on prejudice and violates the civil or human rights of any individual, then that is *discrimination*. An employer who has a prejudice against Asian Americans as managers, hurtful as it may seem, simply has a personally held negative attitude. When the employer refuses to hire or to promote any qualified Asian Americans as managers, then discrimination has taken place. When discriminatory behaviors are acted out in an organized manner at the systemwide or societal level, a situation of *oppression* has occurred. The happenings of discrimination and oppression have forced the situation beyond personal virtue and then become legal, social, and civic concerns.

Although family-health-centered practice uses the strength perspective, it also recognizes the reality of problems and weakness within individuals and social systems. Among these deficiencies are the unjust social systems and human networks that deny people full participation and opportunities for betterment and actualization. Advocacy and empowerment are inherently part of the family health practice.

Similar to the preventive medical health approach, an increasing number of human service professionals are focusing on detecting and addressing risk factors that may negatively affect the quality of life of clients. Risk factors relate to the individual, the family, and their environment, such as peers, school, community, and society. Children who live in families or communities where cigarette smoking is prevalent are at higher risk for the possible health damages caused by secondhand smoke. Similarly, children who live in high crime areas have an increased likelihood of being victims of crime and violence.

## POLICY AND PLANNING

Although the United States does not have a defined family policy, social policy at the local, state, and federal level affects every aspect of our family lives. Close to social work practice are the welfare and public policies such as child care, family planning, housing, employment, income maintenance, domestic violence interventions, child abuse services, health and mental health care, elderly services, and disability. These social policies and their associated programs evolve over time as the result of changing social needs, social philosophy, and the political processes. Franklin and Jordan (1999) provide an overview of major federal social policies and programs that have special relevance in working with families. Their summary serves as the organizing framework for our discussions on policy and planning in this section.

### *Income Maintenance Programs*

The United States has a variety of income maintenance programs. They have been the subjects of many criticisms and congressional revisions; however, they are the fundamental programs that support families. Basically, income maintenance programs include (1) social insurance programs, and (2) public assistance programs.

#### *Social Insurance Programs*

Social insurance programs are comprised of Old Age, Survivors, and Disability Insurance (OASDI, commonly referred to as Social Security); Unemployment Compensation (UC); and Workers' Compensation. Social insurance programs have been the main programs for reducing poverty as well as the major income sources for many American families. In addition to the fact that the implementation of these programs is far from flawless and less than well coordinated, the nature and structure of these programs have also been controversial. Minimum wage standards, gender and ethnic inequity in contributing and receiving support, the pay-as-you-go financing format, and young workers versus retired workers and their spouses are only portions of the ongoing national debates on social insurance programs.

## Public Assistance Programs

Public assistance programs include Supplemental Security Income (SSI), Temporary Assistance to Needy Families (TANF), and General Assistance (GA). Public assistance programs provide cash support to needy individuals and families who have met certain criteria. The 1996 Personal Responsibility and Work Opportunity Reconciliation Act has restructured these federal assistance programs and has posed new challenges for needy families, social workers, and society.

## *Nutrition Programs*

Nutrition policies and programs include the Food Stamp Program; Special Supplemental Nutrition Program for Women, Infants, and Children (WIC); Nutrition Program for Children (school lunch programs); and Nutrition Program for Older Americans (Meals on Wheels).

The Food Stamp Program provides food coupons for purchasing food products. According to the United States Department of Agriculture (USDA) 2000 Budget Summary, in 1999 18.2 million people participated in the food stamp program at a cost of more than $18 billion. Many of the participants are elderly, have disabilities, or have incomes below or near the poverty level. The 1996 welfare reform restricts legal immigrants' eligibility until they become U.S. citizens. New legislations, however, have proposed to restore food stamp benefits to approximately 5,000 elderly immigrants and to 85,000 adults living with eligible legal immigrant children if they entered the United States before August 22, 1996.

The WIC program is a health promotion program that gives nutritional supports to low-income pregnant mothers and their infants and children up to the age of five. It has been credited with enhancing pregnancy outcomes and decreasing medical costs for these families. WIC supplements these households' food resources with vouchers, which can be redeemed for specified foods including milk, eggs, cheese, fruit juices, cereal, and infant formula. In addition to these food supplements, WIC provides nutrition education and linkages to other important health and social services. In 1998, the program budget was slightly over $4 billion and served more than 8 million (8,042,758) women, infants, and children (USDA, 1998). Approximately 47 percent of all infants born in the United States are WIC beneficiaries. The program has contributed to better birth outcomes and reductions in childhood anemia, key indicators of the health of America's children (USDA, 2000).

With a budget of about $10 billion in 1999 (USDA, 2000), the national school lunch, school breakfast, summer food service, special milk, and child and adult care food programs ensure that eligible low-income students receive free or reduced-cost meals and nutrition that meet the Dietary Guidelines for Americans. Preschool and school-aged children in participating schools as well as in child care settings can receive these subsidized meals.

Meals on Wheels and its associated programs at centers for the elderly provide more than meals services to eligible elderly, disabled, or other homebound individuals. The programs help maintain important human and social contacts between service recipients and the service providers who, in many cases, are community volunteers.

### *Housing*

Having a secure and safe living environment is a basic human need. Federally funded housing projects provide housing for low-income families, and Section 8 certificates and housing voucher programs subsidize eligible families to rent privately owned living quarters. Over the years, the term *housing projects* has come to carry the insinuation of drugs, crime, and unsafe environments. In recent years, the federal government has taken on the task of improving both the image and the reality of public housing through redevelopment and community enhancement efforts. Since the mid-1990s, the establishment of empowerment zones and enterprise communities has provided the basis for funding and other supports to a small number of communities to bring about positive change and growth.

In spite of all these efforts toward housing from the different levels of government, and the help of a booming economy in the 1990s, decent and affordable housing is still lacking for many low-income families and individuals. Homelessness, compounded by many psychosocial factors, has been a major social problem—one that has increasingly affected women and children.

The National Law Center on Homelessness and Poverty (1999) estimates that over 700,000 people are homeless on any given night, and up to 2 million people experience homelessness during one year. The U.S. Conference of Mayors (1998) surveyed homelessness in thirty cities and found that children under the age of eighteen accounted for 25 percent of the urban homeless population. They also found that families comprised 38 percent of the homeless population. Shinn and Weitzman (1996) contend that families with children are the fastest-growing segment of the homeless population and constitute approximately 40 percent of people who become homeless. Vissing (1996) reports that families, single mothers, and children make up the largest group of people who are homeless in rural areas.

The National Coalition for the Homeless (2000) reports that among the homeless population, many are ethnic minorities, victims of domestic violence, veterans, and individuals with mental illness and/or drug addiction problems. The U.S. Conference of Mayors (1998) reports the ethnic composition as 49 percent African American, 32 percent Caucasian, 12 percent Hispanic, 4 percent Native American, and 3 percent Asian. They also found domestic violence to be the main cause for homelessness. Approximately 40 percent of homeless men have served in the armed forces, as compared to 34 percent of the general adult male population (Rosenheck, Leda, and Frisman, 1996). About 20 to 25 percent of the single adult homeless population suffers from some form of severe and persistent mental illness (Kegel, Burnam, and Baumohl, 1996).

## *Health Care*

Medicaid is an entitlement program that makes health care services available to poor families and to individuals who do not have health insurance. Although the criteria for eligibility may differ from state to state, the establishment of "medical necessity" is often the essential requirement for eligibility. According to the U.S. Census Bureau 1996 Statistical Abstract, Medicaid is the largest public assistance program, serving approximately 35 million persons at a cost of $144 billion in 1994 (Franklin and Jordan, 1999, p. 363). Medicaid pays for any essential health care services including the costly but important long-term, custodial nursing home, and home health care for many elderly and disabled individuals.

Medicare is a social insurance program funded through Social Security (OASDI) taxes and Medicare tax on payroll. Elderly persons age sixty-five or older and eligible persons with disabilities can receive support for certain health care services, after they have met the requirements of deductible and copayment. Medicare does not pay for all the medical expenses, and many participants buy supplemental policies to cover expenses such as long-term and custodial care.

## *RESEARCH AND PRACTICE EVALUATION*

Social workers are trained to skillfully ask important and relevant questions that may bring about new insight and change. However, social workers have not been particularly active in questioning the effectiveness and quality of their professional interventions. More important, the critical question arises as to whether social work practices are based on sound theories and are grounded in objective as well as subjective data that support the validity of the practice.

Social work research and practice evaluation are systematic inquiries that provide process, outcome, and impact data for service improvement and knowledge development. Process evaluation collects data that answer questions such as the following: Did we do what we set out to do? What have we accomplished? or How did we get it done? Such evaluation involves the report of quantitative information on the logistics and procedural accomplishments as well as the completion of tasks. Attendance records, number of clients served, units of contacts, and many other "bean-counting" activities are examples of process evaluation and data collection.

During the termination and transition stages of the helping relationship, social workers are mindful about the need to evaluate the successes and shortcomings of the helping process. These evaluations do more than just process information; they often involve the very important question, How well did we do? The end results or outcomes of the social work intervention reflect the extent of successes or shortcomings. These are the outcome evaluation and data that measure the extent of change or the qualitative change. Examples of such data include the success rate of using cognitive-behavioral therapy to treat depression among refugee women, the percentage decrease of school dropouts among students in a mentoring program, and the changes of sense of self-efficacy among residents in a housing project.

The inquiry of the often long-range and accumulative effects of social work intervention is referred to as the impact evaluation and data. It attempts to give answers to the cynical but important question of, So what? Impact evaluation addresses the long-term goals and purpose of social work interventions.

A physically abusive father who attends weekly therapeutic group meetings (process) along with biweekly individual counseling (process) for a year (process) has learned to control his anger (outcome) and decrease his alcohol use (outcome). He also has come to a new realization of his responsibilities toward his children, spouse, and extended family (outcome). These insights have led him to become a more caring person for his family and his community (impact).

Family health social work practitioners base their practice on ongoing evaluations that bring about continuous improvement for the practice, theories, and the knowledge base. From exploratory study to descriptive and experimental study, different research designs allow family health practitioners to implement a variety of appropriate practice evaluations. Family health practitioners should also note the utilities of the single-subject design and its contribution toward practice evaluation.

## A CHECKLIST FOR FAMILY-HEALTH–CENTERED INTERVENTIONS

Family health social work practice should be grounded in its adopted theories, include important content areas in the intervention considerations, and apply appropriate skills in the implementation and evaluation of interventions. Chapter 1 reviews the theoretical bases for family-health–centered social work practice. This chapter discusses critical issues related to the important content areas. Chapter 3 proposes a framework for the application of appropriate intervention skills.

The checklist in Figure 2.2 outlines the major issues from the first three chapters of this book (Section I) and serves as a framework that facilitates the design of family-health–centered interventions. Social work practitioners could use this checklist as a reminder or framework for the development and implementation of family-health–centered interventions. The left column lists major areas of concern

| Areas of Concern | Descriptions of Relevance and Implications for Interventions | Skills and Resources |
|---|---|---|
| I. Relevance to family-health–centered practice | | |
|   A. Theoretical considerations and applications | | |
|     1. Ecosystem perspectives | | |
|     2. Developmental theories | | |
|     3. Social constructionist perspectives | | |
|     4. Family practice theories | | |
|     5. Other relevant practice models (e.g., crisis interventions, life model, cognitive-behavioral therapy, etc.) | | |
|   B. Practice content areas considerations | | |
|     1. Human behaviors and social environment: developmental and person-in-environments | | |
|     2. Diversity and cultural competency | | |
|     3. Values and ethical practice | | |
|     4. Concerns for populations at risk, as well as economic and social justice issues | | |
|     5. Policy and planning considerations and developments | | |
|     6. Research and practice evaluation | | |
| II. Levels of intervention and integration | | |
|   A. Individual or microlevel | | |
|   B. Family, group, or mezzolevel | | |
|   C. Community, society, organization, or macrolevel | | |
|   D. Multilevel integration and holistic considerations | | |
| III. Intervention approaches | | |
|   A. Assessment and diagnostic impressions | | |
|   B. Source of problems and symptomatic manifestations | | |
|   C. Theory- and practice-informed intervention strategies and skills | | |
| IV. Evaluation | | |

FIGURE 2.2. Framework for Designing Family-Health–Centered Interventions

that should be considered in any family-health–centered practice. Relevant information about the client(s) should then be listed in the right column.

## *GENERALIST, ADVANCED GENERALIST, SPECIALIZED CONCENTRATIONS, OR FAMILY HEALTH SOCIAL WORK*

Pardeck and colleagues (1998) discuss the differences among generalist, advanced generalist, and family health practice. These distinctions are necessary not only to single out the uniqueness of the family health practice but also to examine the trends of graduate social work education. Nevertheless, more exploration and delineation are productive in reaching a better appreciation of the distinctiveness and interrelatedness of these practice orientations.

In many social work practice situations, social workers use metaphors to help clients as well as themselves to grasp meaning, to understand problems, or to visualize goals and outcomes. The following is a metaphor using cooking school training to better understand the distinctions among various practice orientations. To prepare someone to be a generalist is similar to training someone to become a cook—a regular cook who is prepared to perform most of the basic tasks in the kitchen. This cook is a jack-of-all-trades and may be a good cook for any family-style restaurant where basic meals from appetizers to entrées and desserts are served.

As this cook has sufficient general, or sometimes specific, cooking experiences, she or he may want to advance by returning to school to become a "better cook." In the case of social work training, this better cook is the advanced generalist: a better and more advanced practitioner. The undergraduate social work training programs in the United States primarily prepare students to become generalists. Similarly, the first or foundation year of most of the master of social work (MSW) programs prepares students to be generalists. The difference between first-year graduate social work training and the undergraduate degree training often lies in the intention that first-year MSW students are preparing to go into the second or concentration year, whereas the undergraduates are preparing to go into the workforce as beginning practitioners.

This better-trained cook is supposed to be "better" and may now be looking to work for a more upscale, specialized, or demanding restaurant. Although this cook knows more about the basics and has extra in-depth understanding of the whole business of cooking, periodically or continuously he or she is asked to explain and demonstrate how and why he or she is "better." This situation is similar to the current discussions on advanced generalists. They are versatile and have broad scope and great depth. Advanced generalists can apply multilevel and multimethod approaches to meet the diverse needs of their clients. Many practitioners have adopted this practice model. Equally, many have voiced their concerns for the lack of focus and lack of clear definitions. Advanced generalists are continuously challenged to clarify their focuses and competency.

Instead, if this regular cook goes to one of the schools that employs a popular specialty training, she or he may become a specialty chef: a French, Italian, Chinese, or Mexican cuisine chef. This chef will be, supposedly, better prepared or very competent in the culinary arts within her or his specialty. The limitations, understandably, are in his or her culinary abilities beyond the chosen specialty. Applying this example to social work is the specialization training in concentrations including health, mental health, clinical practice, aging, policy and planning, or planning and administration. Students trained in these specialized concentrations have the in-depth understanding of the subject matter and the mastery of skills to competently accomplish the assigned special tasks. Among their limitations are the restricted considerations and interventions to meet clients of diverse needs.

A family health social worker is like a "head chef" with a mission. As a chef, she or he is able to prepare delicious and/or gourmet meals. As a head chef, she or he knows how to manage a team of chefs and staff to run an effective operation. She or he also knows how to discuss with clients their special culinary needs that may include a big wedding banquet, catered birthday brunch, company New Year celebration, open house, or a unique picnic basket for two. Not only does the head chef know how to prepare a variety of appropriate, high quality culinary productions, he or she also has the ability to recruit, market, assess, plan, organize, and deliver the products. In addition, she or he would call on the supplementary resources available in the market and in the community to meet the client's needs. The head chef aims to do more than cook well or provide a specialty treat. He or she wants to ensure that this is a healthy, balanced, comprehensive, and fulfilling experience—an experience that not only makes sense to the clients, but also meets their various needs and well-being.

A family health social work graduate student is trained to develop generalist skills during the foundation year in the graduate program. The student carries this set of skills, along with the generalist perspectives and initial understanding of family health practice, into the concentration year. The student's knowledge and skills of family health practice are further developed during studies, including field practicum and subsequent post-MSW practices. As a family health social worker, she or he serves clients in many roles that may range from being a clinician, a broker, or an advocate, to being an agency administrator. Among the constants in his or her practice is a focus on promoting the holistic well-being of the family and its members. To achieve that end, the family health social worker may employ a variety of theories, approaches, or skills that are culturally and developmentally appropriate. She or he integrates the family health practice orientation and skills with other preferred models and skills to form her or his own eclectic practice style.

From a cook, to a better cook, French chef, or head chef, social work practice and education have engaged in the ongoing process of evolution and reinvention. Roles include the friendly visitor, the caseworker, the group worker, the community organizer, the radical social worker, the therapist, the administrator, the generic social worker, the generalist, the advanced generalist, the clinician, and possibly the family health social worker. Just as the social work profession values and celebrates human diversity, the profession also promotes and merits unique and well-developed practice models and theories.

## *FUTURE DIRECTIONS*

According to Yuen (1999), the properties and uniqueness of the family health approach will be better understood as it further evolves. Based on Johnson's (1995) framework on social work practice, the following are guidelines for the future development of the family health approach:

1. As a response to concern, the family health approach addresses common human needs. Attention is given to human growth and development; human diversity; related social policy and research issues; and the utilization of ecosystem, social constructionist, and other family-centered perspectives.
2. As a developing approach, it will evolve within the professional social work practice context and the social welfare service environment. The development of the family health approach should be guided by social work values and should adhere to the social work professional code of ethics.
3. As a creative blending of knowledge, values, and skills, the family health approach will evolve and develop its linkages to other social work theories and approaches. Ongoing inquiries of the appropriateness and adequacy of its technology are necessary and desirable. This includes the further identification of the approach's descriptive and prescriptive practice skills.
4. As a social work process, the family health approach promotes holistic health and well-being through a problem-solving approach, utilizing strength perspectives, empowerment, and the exploration of meaningful realities for the individuals and families as well as the profession.
5. As an intervention into human transactions, family health social work practice focuses on the dynamic of the interplays among individuals, families, and related ecosystems. It is a theory-informed, multilevel approach that recognizes the importance and the impacts of human diversity, social justice, and at-risk populations.
6. Most important, family health social work practice is a goal-oriented intervention approach that aims at achieving the well-being of the family and its members.

## REFERENCES

Abbott, E. (1919). The social caseworker and the enforcement of industrial legislation. In *Proceedings of the National Conference on Social Work, 1918* (pp. 310-317). Chicago: Rogers and Hall.

DuBois, B. and Miley, K. (1996). *Social work: An empowering profession.* Boston, MA: Allyn & Bacon.

Franklin, C. and Jordan, C. (1999). *Family practice: Brief systems methods for social work.* Pacific Grove, CA: Brooks/Cole.

Johnson, L. (1995). *Social work practice: A generalist approach,* Fifth edition. Boston, MA: Allyn & Bacon.

Kegel, P., Burnam, M., and Baumohl, J. (1996). The causes of homelessness. In J. Baumohl (Ed.), *Homelessness in America* (pp. 24-23). Phoenix, AZ: Oryx Press.

The National Coalition for the Homeless. (2000). Available online: <http://www.nationalhomeless.org>.

National Law Center on Homelessness and Poverty (1999). *Out of sight—Out of mind? A report on anti-homeless laws, litigation, and alternatives in 50 United States cities.* Washington, DC: Author.

Pardeck, J. T., Yuen, F. K. O, Daley, J., and Hawkins, K. (1998). Social work assessment and intervention through family health practice. *Family Therapy, 25*(1), 25-39.

Rosenheck, R., Leda, C., and Frisman, L. (1996). Homeless veterans. In J. Baumohl (Ed.), *Homelessness in America* (pp. 97-108). Phoenix, AZ: Oryx Press.

Shinn, M. and Weitzman, B. (1996). Homeless families are different. In J. Baumohl (Ed.), *Homelessness in America* (pp. 109-122). Phoenix, AZ: Oryx Press.

U.S. Conference of Mayors (1998). *A status report on hunger and homelessness in America's cities: 1998.* Washington, DC: Author.

U.S. Department of Agriculture (USDA) (1998). *WIC participant and program characteristics: 1998 executive summary.* Available online: <http://www.fns.usda.gov/oane/MENU/Published/WIC/FILES/PC98sum.htm>.

U.S. Department of Agriculture (USDA) (2000). *USDA FY 2001, budget summary.* Available online: <http://www.usda.gov/agency/obpa/Budget-Summary/2001/text.htm#fns>.

Vissing, Y. (1996). *Out of sight, out of mind: Homeless children and families in small town America.* Lexington: The University Press of Kentucky.

Yuen, F. O. (1999). The properties of family health approach. In J. Pardeck and F. Yuen (Eds.), *Family health: A holistic approach to social work practice* (pp. 17-28). Westport, CT: Auburn House.

Chapter 3

# Intervention Strategies of the Family Health Perspective

Gregory J. Skibinski

In today's society in which busy family members have multiple roles, it has become common for families to experience difficulties in everyday life. The simpler times of an agrarian economy, neighborhood churches, representational politics, and stay-at-home moms have been replaced by an international economy, televangelists, presidential investigations, and many dual-career families who need full-time day care and a sport utility vehicle to chauffeur the kids to soccer practice. Consequently, today's family members experience more stress than their predecessors.

"Because of the transactional nature of human interaction, understanding of that environment and its impact is essential for effective service" (Johnson, 1989, p. 241). Social workers embrace the person-in-environment perspective and typically have a broader intervention strategy than do other helping professionals. That perspective leads to more accurate diagnostic impressions and comprehensive treatment approaches. For example, say a female client reports stress as the presenting problem. A psychiatrist who sees this client may diagnose the condition as an anxiety disorder and prescribe a mild sedative. A psychologist would probably diagnose the client similarly and might utilize behavioral or cognitive therapy in treatment. A social worker would probably have a similar diagnostic impression, but the treatment is more likely to isolate the source of the problem.

For example, the social worker might assist the stressed woman and her children by arranging a move to a larger apartment so she does not have to share a bedroom with her three restless children. Perhaps she would need to move from the top floor to the first floor of the housing project, where she can more scrupulously monitor her children's play. The social worker might also help the client find a less stressful job, or one with better wages.

Although prescription medicines, counseling, and coping strategies are acceptable treatments for this woman's condition, they do not focus on her overall situation. Such treatments focus on the manifestations rather than the source of the problem—a stressful environment. "To be maximally effective, interventions, of course, must be directed to all systems that are critical to a given problem system" (Hepworth and Larsen, 1993, p. 17). A broader intervention may include, ultimately, the creation of a neighborhood not-for-profit pharmacy or involve health care advocacy with state legislators. Further, treating manifestations without addressing the source of the problem may result in symptom substitution. For example, if stress triggers a person's smoking, the smoking cessation classes should include techniques of stress management or, if possible, the stress should be eliminated. Unless the source of the problem is addressed, the person may substitute overeating for smoking.

In addition, some problems may require the assistance of other professionals (e.g., physicians, lawyers, local politicians), may take long to accomplish (e.g., developing adequate day care in the neighborhood), or simply be intractable (e.g., a terminal illness). A two-pronged treatment approach is necessary. If at all possible, the social worker should eliminate the source of the problem while simultaneously supporting and maintaining the integrity of the family with coping strategies at various levels. The social worker could take on the role of therapist, advocate, or broker. For example, for an unemployed worker, the social worker might first try to get the client's job back, help file for unemployment or workers' compensation, arrange for updated skills training, or arrange for a transfer to a new department or plant. Simultaneously, the social worker might provide counseling or enlist the help of a psychiatrist for antidepressant drugs, a psychologist for psychotherapy, and refer the client to a job counseling service and a support group. All strategies focus on maintaining the interdependence of family members on each other.

Sections II and III of this book provide case studies based on real situations, with comprehensive diagnostic and treatment packages (and the skills necessary to accomplish and evaluate the treatment goals) for a range of different problems. The case studies are developed from the practice of a professional or licensed family health social worker. The author(s) then analyze and synthesize that case study from a family health perspective according to the following topics:

1. Assessment and diagnostic impressions
2. Identification of problem sources and manifestations
3. Intervention strategies and skills to eliminate both sources and manifestations of the problems
4. Strategies to evaluate intervention

These four topics are discussed in more detail in the following section.

## *ASSESSMENT AND DIAGNOSTIC IMPRESSIONS*

In assessing any family, it is important that the social worker gather information from various sources, especially from the client and family members. Dissimilar to traditional models of assessment such as the medical model, a family health assessment by the social worker is guided by the social constructivist perspective. With that perspective, people interpret issues, ideas, and activities from their own frame of reference based on their understanding, beliefs, and life experiences. Those interpretations affect their construction of reality. For example, if a client defines a lesbian partner as a family member, the social worker must respect that interpretation and treat that couple as a family. Sometimes, however, the social worker must correct faulty perceptions. For example, embezzlement is still a crime even if the bankrupt employee needs the money for Christmas presents.

Further, unlike most other helping professionals, social workers often make home visits and may actually witness the client's living arrangements and circumstances. In viewing the client's environment, the social worker can tap into a rich new source of information unavailable to other professionals. The information not only provides another source of material but also provides background and texture to the client's presenting and real problems. That person-in-environment perspective is what distinguishes social work from the other professions and helps social workers make more comprehensive assessments (Pardeck and Skibinski, 1997).

Consistent with the person-in-environment perspective is a multidimensional assessment. For example, the psychiatrist might focus on the biochemical makeup of a client's brain; the psychologist might focus on the mind through the person's thoughts, actions, and emotions; and a social worker also must focus on the person's family, relationships, use of institutions (e.g., school), and overall environment (e.g., economic situation, family health policies, neighborhood). To successfully assess strengths and weaknesses, a social worker must evaluate a family multidimensionally.

## *Dimensional Assessment of Family and Family Members*

Although a unidimensional assessment might seem sufficient for most problems, often the problems are more complex. Depression, for example, is an affective disorder. However, according to the *Diagnostic and Statistical Manual of Mental Disorders,* Fourth Edition (American Psychiatric Association, 1994), a major depressive episode is characterized by a number of manifestations that might include a depressed mood (affective dimension), indecisiveness (cognitive dimension), insomnia (psychobiological dimension), psychomotor retardation (behavioral and psychobiological dimensions), and social impairment (environmental dimension).

At least five dimensions require assessment: cognitive, affective, behavioral, psychobiological, and environmental. The cognitive dimension, of course, is the indicator of what family members are thinking. Assessment questions from the social worker can be rather direct for this area, although many clients give responses that outline their beliefs instead. According to the social constructivist perspective, clients act on beliefs as if they were facts—defining their reality and guiding their actions. Their beliefs must be respected, and intervention should proceed accordingly.

Equally important is the need for social workers to ascertain how family members feel about a certain issue or situation. Their feelings are often intertwined with their beliefs. Similarly, families also have a set of core values and traditions that transmit feelings to their children. For example, white supremacists might transmit their values through their words and actions. All families, whether intentionally or unintentionally, transmit values to other family members.

Behavioral assessment may be the most important dimension to assess. Most family members do not get into trouble for thinking about domestic violence or for hating someone. It is the action that often causes the person and the family to be referred to the social worker. Behaviors are often readily observable, recordable, and more difficult to hide. Behavioral assessments, therefore, are usually objective, although the reasons for the actions are sometimes speculative. For example, crying is easy to document, but the reason for the crying may be difficult to identify. (Is the child sad, stressed, or in need of a nap?) An assessment that begins with behavioral measures must expand to include other dimensions to ensure accuracy.

In the psychobiological dimension, the social worker assesses how the person's thoughts affect his or her body. For example, being overworked might cause stress. That stress might be manifested in stomach ulcers, nervous tics, or other activities such as pacing. It will have a ripple effect on the family. For example, "Don't bother Dad with your homework tonight. He has a headache from a hard day at work."

The family and its members must also be assessed in their environmental dimension from an ecosystem perspective. The ecosystem perspective is very broad, as it includes intrafamilial relationships, other groups, the neighborhood, and the larger community (e.g., city, state, country, and the world at large). It might seem that the environmental dimension is too large to have an impact on any one person or family, but it can. For example, the global economy has an impact on the U.S. stock market, and that has an impact on a family's well-being, especially if the family's income or retirement is tied to those funds. In family health practice, the two most significant dimensions are the behavioral and environmental dimensions, as they dictate family members' interactions with the family and outside world.

## *Data-Gathering Techniques*

Traditionally, social workers have used interviews as their main assessment tool. This method has limitations, as interviewers often focus on behavioral and affective information. Many other methods of gathering information exist, including already-collected data sources (e.g., school or medical records), behavioral evidence (the number of empty beer bottles in an alcoholic's garbage), or measurement instruments such as those developed by Walter Hudson (e.g., the Generalized Contentment Scale). Social workers need to gather information from any available sources. Many of these assessment tools and techniques can be used throughout the intervention period and for followup (see Daley, 1999).

In the past two decades, social workers have developed a number of instruments to measure sources and manifestations of problems in many areas. Although most of the instruments evaluate personal and interpersonal well-being, some of the measures evaluate social problems and other macrolevel needs. One such author is Walter Hudson (1982), whose instrument package *(The Clinical Measurement Package: A Field Manual)* was the impetus for many authors to develop assessment tools. Hudson has now more than tripled his number of assessment instruments. Shortly after Hudson's publication, Corcoran and Fischer (1987) pulled together many existing assessment instruments from disparate sources. In 1994 they published a second edition (Fischer and Corcoran, 1994), more than doubling the volume of their earlier work. The latter work includes many instruments to objectively measure couples and families. For example, their book includes the Family Assessment Device and the Self-Report Family Instrument, among others.

Finally, social workers need cooperation and information from other professionals and professional agencies. Sources include a mental status exam from psychiatrists, psychological evaluations, medical and dental records, or school records on the children. Conversely, social workers can request evaluations by other professionals.

## *PROBLEM SOURCES AND MANIFESTATIONS*

If at all possible, the family health social worker should identify and eliminate the source of the problem. Although that directive may seem both obvious and simplistic, it is often neither. In other professions, most obviously the medical profession, treating symptoms alone, or even introducing side effects (iatrogenic manifestations), appears normative. Treating hypertension with medication, rather than relieving the person's stress, is one example of treating the symptoms without eliminating the source. Hypertensive medication may also cause erectile dysfunction. The parallel situation for social workers is to provide symptomatic relief for their clients through the employment of coping strategies. Although acceptable for intractable problems, or temporary relief for long-term conditions (e.g., changing eligibility requirements for welfare recipients), elimination of the source of the problem is the only permanent solution to many family problems.

For example, little long-term good is achieved in keeping a family on Temporary Assistance to Needy Families (TANF) if the potential breadwinner wants to learn a skill or obtain an education. Determining whether the presenting problem is merely a manifestation of a larger problem or the actual source of the problem is a function of the social worker's education, professional judgment, and quality of the assessment.

## INTERVENTION SKILLS TO ELIMINATE BOTH SOURCES AND MANIFESTATIONS

The focus of a family health social worker must be on the well-being of the family, which requires a mix of interventions at all levels (micro, mezzo, and macro). Microskills such as attending, communicating, questioning, confronting, brokering, and mediating are a necessary part of intervention. Macroskills are also necessary, as the family may have trouble negotiating the complexities of social institutions (e.g., schools, social service agencies, courts). Intervention skills may include budgeting, negotiating, social reform, policy development, mediating, or influencing decision makers. In family health practice, mezzolevel interventions can be divided into family counseling and noncounseling interventions.

### *Family Counseling*

Once the contributions of individual family members are determined, an assessment of the family must be made. A number of issues must be addressed, such as family homoeostasis, rules, boundaries, power, decision making, roles, communications, and other dimensions (Hepworth, Rooney, and Larsen, 1997). Each family has its own level of equilibrium. Family history, culture, member needs, and the current dilemma influence that level. To maintain equilibrium, the family develops roles for each member, which may or may not be consistent with the current culture. In dysfunctional families, a member may have overstepped boundaries or violated the power structure or decision-making protocol of the family. Often, a lack of communication exists. For some dysfunctional families, the intervention strategy of choice may be family counseling.

Numerous approaches to family counseling are taken. Goldenberg and Goldenberg (1996) identify thirty-five theories, categorizing the theories by constructs into eight models: Psychodynamic, Experiential/Humanistic, Bowenian, Structural, Communication/Strategic, Milan/Systemic, Behavioral/Cognitive, and Postmodern. Barnhill (1979) summarizes family theories by process variables. He finds four main processes, each with two diametrically opposing characteristics. Barnhill's findings, referenced to the major theorist or theoretical school (significant authors and theories in parenthesis) follow.

## Barnhill's Summary of Family Theories by Process Variables

1. *Identity processes* of the family, which include members'
   a. *individuation* (vs. enmeshment: Bowen, family systems; Boszormenyi-Nagy, contextual; Whitaker, symbolic-experiential; and Wynne).
   b. *mutuality* (vs. isolation: Whitaker, symbolic-experiential; and Wynne).
2. *Change* is comprised of
   a. *flexibility* (vs. rigidity: Haley and Jackson, communication/strategic; Ackerman, psychoanalytic; and others).
   b. *stability* (vs. disorganization: Jackson, communication/strategic).
3. *Information processing* is subdivided into
   a. *clear perception* (vs. distorted perception: Ackerman, psychoanalytic; Bowen, family systems; Boszormenyi-Nagy, contextual; and Wynne).
   b. *clear communication* (vs. distorted communication: Bateson et al.; Jackson, communication/strategic; and Satir, human validation).
4. *Role structuring,* which includes
   a. *role reciprocity* (vs. role conflict: Jackson, communication/strategic; Spiegel; Lidz; and Tharp and Otis).
   b. *clear generational boundaries* (vs. breached generational boundaries: Haley, communication/strategic; Lidz; and Minuchin, structural).

These family counseling theories can be helpful for families who exhibit isolated or focused problems as determined in the assessment. For example, if communication between family members is the family's only problem, family counseling using Jackson's or Satir's theories may be quite appropriate. However, most problems are not so focused, as problems often occur in other systems. Those problems require other intervention strategies.

## *Noncounseling Intervention*

Aside from problems that necessitate family counseling, other problems occur that may necessitate noncounseling interventions, such as teaching the family problem-solving skills, assertiveness training, and stress relief. Many of the group skills and theories apply because families are a special type of group. Those mezzolevel practice skills include, but are not limited to, brokering, mediating, facilitating, decision making, and coordinating. The group theories of Yalom, Vinter, Glasser, Garvin, Schwartz, and others are pertinent.

What differentiates family health intervention strategies from other orientations, especially generalist practice, is the focus on families. Whatever needs to be done with a case, the focus must be on family improvement, even if much of the intervention is directed at one or more family members. For example, in a family, alcoholism requires an enabler, and treatment may first focus on the alcoholic and the enabler, not on the entire family. The other family members may participate as needed and when willing. Ultimately, the family benefits.

## STRATEGIES TO EVALUATE INTERVENTION

Although many ways are available to evaluate the outcome of interventions with families, such as the social worker's professional judgment or the client's personal satisfaction, it is most important that the measure be valid and reliable. In general, objective, quantifiable measures are preferable. In the social sciences, that often means behavioral measures or the use of instruments. For example, behaviors are easily counted by frequency, duration, interval, and magnitude. *Frequency* is simply the number of times a behavior occurs (e.g., the child cries every time he or she sees a dog; the number of assaults in a neighborhood). *Duration* is the length of time a behavior occurs (e.g., the child cried for five minutes; the mayor has opposed the project for seven years). *Interval* is the time between the presentation of some stimulus and a behavior (e.g., the child was stunned at first by the dog's presence and began to cry about ten seconds later; the lag time between identified need and policy implementation). Finally, *magnitude* is the intensity of a behavior (e.g., it was the loudest crying ever heard from a four-year-old child; the shouts of the demonstrators were deafening).

Instruments, which are described in more detail in the assessment section of this chapter, are also useful as postassessment evaluation tools. They are most helpful in converting subjective indicators into more objective measures (e.g., the scaling of attitudes toward family members or issues).

Regardless of the type of objective measures used, the clinician can put such objective measures into graphic form. Graphing is especially helpful as it supplies information in more than one medium (numerical and pictorial) and is more easily understood by family members. Because it demonstrates trends, the graph may serve a motivating function as well.

Finally, to increase the scientific integrity of the decision-making process, single-system designs should be used whenever possible. They are relatively simple to use, and the techniques are often taught in research courses of accredited schools of social work. For more information on intervention evaluation strategies, see Alter and Evens, 1990; Bloom, Fischer, and Orme, 1995; Campbell, 1988; Fischer and Corcoran, 1994; Gabor and Grinnell, 1994; Magura, Moses, and Jones, 1987; Nugent, Sieppert, and Hudson, 2001; and Mattaini, 1993.

Alternately, evaluation of a social worker's family health interventions may require a qualitative approach. For example, when evaluations are done in a natural setting in which it is difficult to manipulate the variables, the evaluation questions are not fully conceptualized, or the focus is on process rather than outcome variables, the use of qualitative evaluation techniques (e.g., participant observation) may be necessary (Tutty, Rothery, and Grinnell, 1996).

# EXAMPLE CASE STUDY AND INTERVENTION TEMPLATE

Many chapters in Sections II and III analyze case studies according to the following template:

1. Assessment and diagnostic impressions
2. Source of the problem and manifestations
   a. Assessing the source of the problem
   b. Manifestations
3. Intervention strategies and activities to eliminate both sources and manifestations
   a. Manifestation relief (e.g., coping strategies)
   b. Source elimination
4. Strategies to evaluate intervention

## Example Case Study

You are a social worker in a family practice clinic in Springfield. Your latest referral is a Mrs. Darlene C., who claims to be anxious. You obtain the following information during your assessment.

Darlene is a thirty-nine-year-old mother of two. She is employed at a local manufacturing plant on first shift as a bookkeeper. Darlene has been married to John, a laborer there, for nineteen years. They have two children, Allen, age seventeen, and Sandy, age seven.

Darlene describes her problem as follows: Until recently, the family had been together but not happy. The husband, John, has a severe drinking problem and although he has been hospitalized for this condition ("forced" he says), he is presently drinking heavily and denies any problems with alcohol. His driver's license was revoked two weeks ago for driving while intoxicated. About two months ago, John's yearly checkup at work revealed that he had early symptoms of cirrhosis of the liver. The physician told Darlene that unless her husband stops drinking immediately, he will die within two years. When their son, Allen, heard the news, he stormed out of the house and took the family car. Five hours later, Darlene got a call from the police department that Allen was being held on the charge of driving while intoxicated. The police found him alone and uninjured in the car after smashing into a yard on the south side of Springfield. Last week, Allen was found guilty of driving while intoxicated and placed on probation. The only condition of probation was that he pays for the damages to the car and the yard ($800 total, to be paid to the clerk of courts in $25 weekly installments). Darlene wants you to monitor the situation.

Darlene describes herself as "nervous." Your assessment confirms her opinion, and you enter a diagnostic impression of anxious depression. Since the root of the problem appears to be the husband's drinking problem, and it seems to affect the entire family, you suggest a comprehensive intervention.

## *Intervention Plan (Abbreviated)*

*Assessment and Diagnostic Impression*

1. Darlene has anxious depression.
2. Darlene is not an assertive person and may be an enabler.
3. John appears to be an alcoholic.
4. John lost his driver's license.
5. Allen must repay damages, attend school, and work his part-time job.
6. Dysfunctional family—alcohol dependence.

*Intervention Activities*

1. The client is experiencing anxious depression and all of its symptoms (e.g., inability to concentrate, fatigue). Social worker will see client weekly for treatment of the depression and monitor progress with the Zung Self-Rating Depression Scale (MANIFESTATION).
2. Lack of assertiveness by client. Assertiveness training classes, held weekly by the local mental health agency suggested. Social worker will administer the Rathus Assertiveness Schedule and utilize results to monitor progress (SOURCE).
3. Husband's drinking behavior. To be monitored only—no intervention, per Darlene's request. Darlene will count and record the number of bottles of beer her husband consumes per day (SOURCE).
4. Social worker to negotiate with the department of transportation for work-related driving privileges. Alternately, enlist local self-help or charitable group to drive John to and from work (MANIFESTATION).
5. Son's reimbursement for damages. Social worker to make a phone call each week to the clerk of court to verify payment (MANIFESTATION).

6. Son's school attendance. Social worker will monitor each day with a phone call to the school's attendance officer (MANIFESTATION).
7. Son's attendance at his part-time job. Operationally defined as twenty hours per week, verified by Allen's weekly paycheck stub (MANIFESTATION).
8. Family treatment (all family members will be encouraged to attend). Especially in areas of (a) identity process, (b) family stability, and (c) clear perception by John (monitored by Family Assessment Device) (SOURCE).

*Evaluation Strategies*

Intervention activities 1, 2, and 8 can be monitored graphically via an instrument score. The three instruments have interpretive guidelines of the levels of depression and assertiveness based on the subject's score. Activity 3 should be monitored by counting and graphing the number of bottles of beer husband John drinks. Activities 5, 6, and 7 can be monitored by a weekly compliance checklist (e.g., comply; did not comply).

## CONCLUSION

The family health perspective makes two significant contributions to the family intervention landscape: first is the use of the whole family as an anchor for the intervention process; second, the perspective is broader in scope than the so-called "talking therapies," which are more likely to be focused on symptom reduction or coping strategies than eliminating the source of the family problem.

## REFERENCES

Alter, C. and Evens, W. (1990). *Evaluating your practice: A guide to self-assessment*. New York: Springer.
American Psychiatric Association (1994). *Diagnostic and statistical manual of mental disorders,* Fourth edition. Washington, DC: Author.
Barnhill, L. R. (1979). Healthy family systems. *The Family Coordinator,* January, pp. 94-100.

Bloom, M., Fischer, J., and Orme, J. (1995). *Evaluating practice: Guidelines for the accountable professional*, Second edition. Englewood Cliffs, NJ: Prentice-Hall.

Campbell, J. A. (1988). Client acceptance of single-system evaluation procedures. *Social Work Research and Abstracts, 24,* 21-22.

Corcoran, K. and Fischer, J. (1987). *Measures for clinical practice: A sourcebook.* New York: The Free Press.

Daley, J. G. (1999). Clinical instruments for assessing family health. In J. T. Pardeck and F. K. O. Yuen (Eds.), *Family health: A holistic approach to social work practice* (pp. 81-99). Westport, CT: Auburn.

Fischer, J. and Corcoran, K. J. (1994). *Measures for clinical practice: A sourcebook,* Second edition. New York: The Free Press.

Gabor, P. A. and Grinnell, R. M. (1994). *Evaluation and quality improvement in the human services.* Needham Heights, MA: Allyn & Bacon.

Goldenberg, I. and Goldenberg, H. (1996). *Family therapy: An overview,* Fourth edition. Pacific Grove, CA: Brooks/Cole.

Hepworth, D. H. and Larsen, J. A. (1993). *Direct social work practice: Theory and skills,* Fourth edition. Pacific Grove, CA: Brooks/Cole.

Hepworth, D. H., Rooney, R. H., and Larsen, J. A. (1997). *Direct social work practice: Theory and skills,* Fifth edition. Pacific Grove, CA: Brooks/Cole.

Hudson, W. W. (1982). *The clinical measurement package: A field manual.* Homewood, IL: The Dorsey Press.

Johnson, L. (1989). *Social work practice: A generalist approach,* Third edition. Needham Heights, MA: Allyn & Bacon.

Magura, S., Moses, B. S., and Jones J. A. (1987). *Assessing risk and measuring change in families: The Family Risk Scales.* Washington, DC: The Child Welfare League of America.

Mattaini, M. A. (1993). *More than a thousand words: Graphics for clinical practice.* Washington, DC: NASW Press.

Nugent, W. M., Sieppert, J. D., and Hudson, W. W. (2001). *Practice evaluation for the 21st century.* Belmont, CA: Wadsworth/Thomson Learning.

Pardeck, J. T. and Skibinski, G. J. (1997). An exploration of the practice orientations of licensed clinical social workers and licensed clinical psychologists. *The Clinical Supervisor, 16*(2), 125-137.

Tutty, L. M., Rothery, M., and Grinnell, R. M. (1996). *Qualitative research for social workers: Phases, steps, and tasks.* Boston, MA: Allyn & Bacon.

# SECTION II:
# FAMILY HEALTH APPROACH IN PRACTICE

Chapter 4

# Child Maltreatment and Family Health Practice

Gregory J. Skibinski

In this chapter, a case of child sexual abuse is discussed from the family health perspective. The family scenario is based on a case encountered in a large Midwestern city. Two sets of intervention strategies are discussed: first, the specific intervention used with this family; and second, the impetus this representative case served as to cause sweeping changes at the macrolevel, which would benefit future victims and their families.

## *ASSESSMENT AND DIAGNOSTIC IMPRESSION*

### *Social History*

The Schutkin family is a traditional family living in a large Midwestern city. The main industry of the town is manufacturing, and many of the residents are blue-collar workers. As with most industrial towns, the city is adapting to the changing economy and is broadening its economic base by becoming more service oriented. Many of the workers are in job training programs or returning to school. Mr. Schutkin is a factory laborer who is rather set in his ways. He is forty-three years old and has been employed on third shift at the same factory since he was twenty-seven. He never aspired to be anything more than what he is. He has been married to Celine, thirty-seven, for the past ten years. It is the a second marriage for both. His first marriage produced no children; Celine's produced a boy (Jeremy, now seventeen) and a girl (Rebecca, now twelve). Both children live in the Schutkin household, and Mr. Schutkin (Paul) did not adopt either of the children. No contact occurs between the biological father and Mrs. Schutkin or the children.

Mrs. Schutkin is also a laborer. She works in light manufacturing and has worked on second shift for her current company for the past fifteen years. As a result of their work schedules, Mr. and Mrs. Schutkin do not see each other much during the week. Because of Mrs. Schutkin's work schedule, most of the housework is left to the rest of the family, and Mr. Schutkin helps with Jeremy and Rebecca's homework. Jeremy has a part-time job at a nearby restaurant chain. He does few of the home chores.

The local division of family services received this case as a potential abuse and neglect case referred by the social worker at Rebecca's school. She noticed a change in Rebecca's attitude, temperament, and behavior in the previous six months. This is the first referral for either of the children with either set of parents. A social worker was dispatched to the Schutkin house within a week of the referral. He interviewed the four family members together and separately.

Based on these interviews, he concluded that Mr. Schutkin had probably molested Rebecca on three separate occasions in the past six months. As no reports were made of digital, oral, or penal penetration, the abuse seemed to be limited to exploratory fondling, a common precursor to intercourse. No referral had been made to a physician, nor has any physician discovered any abusive symptomology during routine examinations. The social worker based his findings on Rebecca's story, her change in mood and behavior, the environmental scenario (the opportunity provided by Mrs. Schutkin's nightly absence from the home and the increased caretaking role by the daughter), and the strain in the marital relationship reported by Mrs. Schutkin. Mr. Schutkin denied any wrongdoing, and Mrs. Schutkin was unaware of any sexual abuse. The case was then referred to a child advocacy center for evaluation. They reported similar findings and also included abuse of alcohol by the father as a contributing factor.

## *PROBLEM SOURCES AND MANIFESTATIONS*

### *Child Sexual Abuse (MANIFESTATION)*

In the Schutkin home, and common in most cases of incest, the abuse is often a symptom of some larger familial problem. In this case, the child sex abuse seems to have occurred because of the combination of alcohol abuse by the father and marital problems of the parents.

## *Pseudomaturity of Rebecca Due to Role Confusion (MANIFESTATION)*

Because of the work schedules of the parents, all family members must assist in household maintenance chores such as cleaning, laundry, and meal preparation. With her brother holding an outside job, most of the evening chores fall to Rebecca and her stepfather. Being a young girl in a traditional family, she feels it necessary to shoulder the burden of the "women's work" to help her employed mother, and to care for her father and brother.

## *Marital Strain (CAUSE)*

Mrs. Schutkin reports marital strain for the past few years based on work schedules, lack of affection, and her husband's drinking.

## *Alcohol Abuse by Mr. Schutkin (CAUSE)*

Mr. Schutkin has an undiagnosed, untreated alcohol-dependence problem that probably dates back to his early twenties.

## *ACTIVITIES TO ELIMINATE BOTH SOURCES AND MANIFESTATIONS*

## *Child Sexual Abuse (MANIFESTATION)*

Assessment and intervention strategies common to the time periods were used. Following the referral, the social worker investigated the case and reported his findings to the police. Rebecca was referred to a victim center for a physical examination and counseling. Some attempts were made to involve the other family members, but Jeremy was not interested, and Mrs. Schutkin was unavailable during non-school hours. Mr. Schutkin was never approached. Aside from the physical examination and counseling, Rebecca was given some tips on fending off future attacks and how to discuss the incident should questions from her peers arise. She received little advice or support from the legal professionals.

*Rationale for Macrointervention*

Based on clinical experience and the professional literature at the time of this case (early 1990s), intrafamilial child sexual abuse was believed to be a symptom of family dysfunction (Finkelhor, 1978; Frude, 1982; Giaretto, 1982; Salter, 1988). Family intervention is the most logical treatment route but rarely occurs if prosecution and imprisonment are pursued because the goals of those systems are punitive, not rehabilitative. Further, traditional prosecutions of child sexual abuse offenders are problematic for many reasons, most notably because convictions are difficult (Eatman and Bulkley, 1986; Harshbarger, Botsford, and Keeler, 1986); sentences are short (MacFarlane and Bulkley, 1982; University of Wisconsin Law School [UWLS], 1986); and offender treatment is unlikely (Eatman and Bulkley, 1986; UWLS, 1986). Although physical separation by imprisonment will temporarily stop the offender from abusing the child, no assurance can be made that once released, the offender will not abuse again, especially without treatment in prison.

Local mental health services, social services, and legal and criminal professionals decided to develop a cooperative, nontraditional strategy for child sexual abuse cases with both a legal and treatment focus. The primary goals guiding the creation and development of such innovative programs are to provide treatment for the victim and his or her family (including siblings and nonoffending caregivers), to rehabilitate the offender, and to minimize system-induced trauma for the child and his or her family (i.e., secondary victimization through testifying) (Berliner and Barbieri, 1984; Colby and Colby, 1987; Gothard, 1987; Higgins, 1988; Koszuth, 1991; MacFarlane and Bulkley, 1982; Ordway, 1983; Skibinski and Esser-Stuart, 1993; Weiss and Berg, 1982; Whitcomb, 1991). The assault and the secondary victimization may be cumulatively damaging. The program, developed as a result of cases similar to this case study, was designed for first-time, intrafamilial child sexual abuse offenders. Apparently, the professionals believed that nonpunitive or minimally punitive programs serve society best by keeping the family intact and the initial assault secret. It was believed to be a good compromise between the victim's and society's right to protection and the victim's, family's, and offender's right to treatment.

## *Actual Program Developed from This Case: Postarraignment (Postplea) Diversion Program*

Rather than arresting the alleged offender, the accused in this case attended a pretrial conference to determine his treatability. If the alleged offender was treatable (could significantly benefit from treatment as judged by the caseworker, the district attorney, and the social worker from the diversion program) and was willing to accept responsibility for the assault, the accused was charged, pled guilty at the initial appearance, and was deferred from further prosecution into the preexisting treatment program (counseling and other mental health and social services). The guilty plea was vacated if the accused successfully completed the treatment program (determined by the professional judgment of the primary therapist of the treatment program). If unsuccessful, the guilty plea was entered and the perpetrator was sentenced as a felon.

A family court (i.e., juvenile court) petition was also filed on behalf of the victims, allowing the victim and family members to receive treatment and various services via court order.

## **Pseudomaturity of Rebecca Due to Role Confusion (MANIFESTATION)**

With Mrs. Schutkin working second shift at the local factory, many of the household duties have fallen onto Rebecca's shoulders. Of course, assuming household chores is a good experience, but Rebecca should not have to take primary responsibility for the work; that responsibility should fall to Mr. Schutkin. The family composed a list of household chores, including names of family members responsible for task completion. The social worker reviewed and adjusted the list in a family meeting. Rebecca's chores were significantly reduced. Mrs. Schutkin agreed to prepare and freeze daily meals in her free time. Removing this context of pseudomaturity was believed to reduce the likelihood of further assaults. The social worker also provided Rebecca with counseling for the assaults and educational material on social and recreational activities appropriate for her age. The parents received similar information. Rebecca was encouraged to spend at least one hour per day after school with her friends.

## *Marital Strain (CAUSE)*

The Schutkins have had long-standing marital problems. They were referred to a family therapist for weekly counseling sessions. Mrs. Schutkin always attended; her husband usually did so.

## *Alcohol Abuse by Mr. Schutkin (CAUSE)*

Mr. Schutkin was not ready to admit that he had a substance abuse problem. Although he was given names, addresses, and meeting dates of the local Alcoholics Anonymous (AA) programs in the area, he was in denial and did not attend any meetings. His drinking patterns were unchanged throughout the course of the social worker's intervention, yet efforts to convince him to seek help continued.

The social worker referred the children to Al-Anon/Alateen and Mrs. Schutkin to Al-Anon.

## **STRATEGIES TO EVALUATE INTERVENTION**

### *Child Sexual Abuse*

To monitor the possibility of ongoing sexual assaults by Mr. Schutkin, the social worker obtained weekly reports via phone from Rebecca's teachers and conducted weekly interviews with Mrs. Schutkin and Rebecca during regular visitations. The social worker provided everyone a list of potential victim characteristics (e.g., change in mood, withdrawal, secrecy). The counselor at the victim center provided similar reports that included her professional opinion on Rebecca's progress in counseling.

### *Pseudomaturity of Rebecca*

A checklist of Rebecca's assigned chores was developed and completed each night before bedtime. Any chores beyond those listed were noted on a separated sheet of paper. Rebecca also listed on that sheet each meal that she, and not her mother, prepared.

On three separate occasions, the social worker provided educational information about age-appropriate activities. Rebecca was given one week to read each set of materials. She complied in each case.

Finally, Rebecca had a checklist for playtime with her neighborhood or school friends. She listed how much time per day was playtime and wrote down the names of her playmates.

## *Marital Strain*

The number of marital counseling sessions for both Mr. and Mrs. Schutkin was tracked through monthly calls to the marriage counselor. Both partners granted the marriage counselor permission to release such information. The marriage counselor also provided professional judgment on the couple's progress. Although some progress was made individually, especially for Mrs. Schutkin, little progress was reported for the couple. Mr. Schutkin's drinking (and subsequent behavior) was considered the major impediment to progress.

Mrs. Schutkin also agreed to complete the Index of Marital Satisfaction instrument (Hudson, 1992) before and after treatment. Little progress was noted.

## *Alcohol Abuse*

Tallies were kept of each family member's attendance of Alcoholics Anonymous, Al-Anon, and Alateen meetings. An attempt was made to have Mr. Schutkin take the Michigan Alcoholism Screening Test (Selzer, 1971). Mr. Schutkin refused. Opinions of Mrs. Schutkin regarding her husband's drinking were routinely received. Mr. Schutkin denied any drinking problem.

## REFERENCES

Berliner, L. and Barbieri, M. K. (1984). The testimony of the child victim of sexual assault. *Journal of Social Issues, 40*(2), 125-137.

Colby, I. and Colby, D. (1987). Videotaping the child sexual-abuse victim. *Social Casework: The Journal of Contemporary Social Work, 68,* 117-121.

Eatman, R. and Bulkley, J. (1986). *Protecting child victim/witnesses: Sample laws and materials.* Washington, DC: American Bar Association.

Finkelhor, D. (1978). Psychological, cultural, and family factors in incest and family sexual abuse. *Journal of Marriage and Family Counseling,* October, 41-48.

Frude, N. (1982). The sexual nature of sexual abuse: A review of the literature. *Child Abuse and Neglect, 6,* 211-223.

Giaretto, H. (1982). *Integrated treatment of child sexual abuse.* Palo Alto, CA: Science and Behavior.

Gothard, S. (1987). The admissibility of evidence in child sexual abuse cases. *Child Welfare, 66*(1), 13-24.

Harshbarger, S., Botsford, M., and Keeler, K. J. (1986). Prosecuting child sexual abuse cases in Middlesex County. *Boston Bar Journal, 30*(2), 6-11.

Higgins, R. B. (1988). Child victims and witnesses. *Law and Psychology Review, 12,* 159-166.

Hudson, W. W. (1992). *The WALMYR Assessment Scales scoring manual.* Tempe, AZ: WALMYR.

Koszuth, A. (1991). Sexually abused child syndrome: *Res ipsa loquitur* and shifting the burden of proof. *Law and Psychology Review, 15* (spring), 277-297.

MacFarlane, K. and Bulkley, J. (1982). Treating child sexual abuse: An overview of current program models. *Social Work and Child Sexual Abuse, 1*(1/2), 69-91.

Ordway, D. P. (1983). Reforming judicial procedures for handling parent-child incest. *Child Welfare, LXII,* 68-75.

Salter, A. C. (1988). *Treating child sex offenders and victims.* Newbury Park, CA: Sage.

Selzer, M. L. (1971). The Michigan Alcoholism Screening Test: The quest for a new diagnostic instrument. *American Journal of Psychiatry, 127,* 89-94.

Skibinski, G. J. and Esser-Stuart, J. E. (1993). Public sentiment toward innovative child sexual abuse intervention strategies: An empirical study of consensus and conflict. *Juvenile and Family Court Journal, 44*(3), 17-26.

University of Wisconsin Law School (UWLS). (1986). *Punish the offender, protect the victim, treat the family.* Madison, WI: Author.

Weiss, E. H. and Berg, R. F. (1982). Child victims of sexual assault: Impact of court procedures. *Journal of the American Academy of Child Psychiatry, 21,* 513-518.

Whitcomb, D. (1991). Improving the investigation and prosecution of child sexual-abuse cases: Research findings, questions, and implications for public policy. In D. D. Knudsen and J. L. Miller (Eds.), *Abused and battered: Social and legal responses to family violence* (pp. 181-190). New York: Aldine de Gruyter.

Chapter 5

# Intervening with Domestic Violence Using the Family Health Perspective

Joan C. McClennen

## *INTRODUCTION*

This case is based on true accounts from women in a shelter for victims of domestic violence. Although the situations of victims vary extensively, the circumstances of this case are not uncommon. Similarities in circumstances include that each of the female victims

1. lived for years with her abusive husband;
2. had at least one child fathered by the abuser;
3. had left the abuser;
4. after being separated, was stalked and abused by her ex-husband;
5. did not receive reprieve from the abuse even though she sought professional help (attorneys, police, welfare, and criminal justice system);
6. still, at least subconsciously, was trying to please her abuser;
7. had at least one child fathered by a boyfriend after her divorce;
8. continued contact with the boyfriend;
9. had no employment skills, housing, or appreciable resources; and
10. wanted to keep her children and stop living in fear.

Using the family health perspective in assessing and intervening with victims of domestic violence, social workers are guided by several underlying theories and approaches (systems theory, ecological approach, and the social constructionist theory). The *systems theory* emphasizes the need to consider the interrelationship and interconnectedness among individuals within the family (Pardeck and Yuen, 1997). Intervention takes place on the micro-, mezzo-, and macro-levels to adequately address the various aspects of the family's health. The *ecological approach* requires the social worker to assume various roles (advocate, broker, mediator) in assuring reciprocal dynamics between the person and the environment throughout the intervention process. The *social constructionist theory* emphasizes people's ability to make sense of their own experiences and the social worker's responsibility to respect the clients' interpretation of events. Identifying and intervening with families experiencing domestic violence requires an alliance between the social worker, the client, and other professionals to effectively alleviate this sensitive social problem. With these theoretical bases, the social worker initiates assessment and intervention processes.

## *SOCIAL WORKER'S INITIAL INTERVIEW WITH RITA*

Rita was referred to the clinical social worker within the domestic violence shelter due to her anxiety about her situation, especially in respect to her children's custody. Rita had recently shown up on the doorstep of the shelter with her three children: Alfred, age ten; Roger, age eight; and Lauren, age six months. Rita was running from her ex-husband and had nowhere to turn. She was admitted to the shelter that evening.

Rita was skeptical yet relatively open and articulate in explaining her past and present situation. At age twenty, she had been "swept off her feet" by her ex-husband, Jack. One week after the marriage, the abuse began. Describing herself as formerly physically fit and attractive, Rita stated she now was overweight and worn.

Jack often became intoxicated and sexually, physically, psychologically, and financially abused Rita. Rita repeatedly stated that she "had" to do what Jack wanted. The abuse escalated in intensity and in frequency.

Rita became pregnant shortly after the marriage. During her pregnancy, Jack would hit her in the abdomen seemingly trying to cause a miscarriage. This happened during both of her first two pregnancies.

She described one incident of sexual abuse that occurred shortly after the birth of her second son, Roger. She had returned home after a difficult delivery. She had stitches from the natural birth. Jack insisted on sexual relations. When she refused, he raped her.

The family barely survived financially. Jack went from job to job; Rita stayed home with the children. At one point they lived in an apartment in which the stove had only one burner working. Although he refused to spend the thirty-eight dollars to fix the stove, Jack insisted his full-course meals be ready upon his return home from work.

Rita had sought help from her family, who encouraged her to leave Jack. She did not elaborate on her family but spoke more about Jack's background. He had been raised in an abusive home in which his father beat him and his siblings. Neither family of origin appeared to be involved with Rita at this time.

Three years ago, Rita divorced Jack; they had joint custody of the two boys. He seldom complied with the child support; Rita lived mainly on welfare.

Periodically, Jack would show up at Rita's house and beat her. At one point the neighbors called the police. By the time the officers arrived, Rita had a bloody nose and was, as happened often in the past, covered with bruises. She said the officers told them that if they had to come to the house again, someone would be arrested. They left, at which time Jack beat Rita even harder for embarrassing him. She said she would never trust the police again.

Within about six months after her divorce, Rita met Kevin, her present boyfriend and the father of Lauren. Rita and Kevin decided to relocate to this state as it was where Kevin was raised. Although Rita and Kevin moved to this state together, they lived in different households. Rita feared that Jack would come to her home and Kevin would either get hurt or get in trouble for hurting Jack.

Eventually, Rita asked Jack to care for the two boys so she could get financially established. During the boys' absence, she became pregnant with Lauren. Rita then decided she wanted the boys to live with her. Jack refused. He would not allow Rita to see the boys except under strict supervision.

Periodically, Rita would hear about the boys through her mother. At one point, her mother called and said Jack was leaving the boys at her house. Rita and Kevin drove to the mother's house and brought the boys to this state.

Although infuriated, Jack told Rita she could keep the boys for a few weeks. He informed her that he had the Federal Bureau of Investigation (FBI) watching her and would have his "connections" take care of her if she did not return the children at the designated date.

While in the care of Rita and Kevin, the boys fought almost constantly, hitting and yelling at each other. Roger seemed to have more extensive behavioral difficulties than Alfred. Roger would scream and defecate in his pants when upset. After one episode of stopping the fighting between the boys, Kevin went into a room with Roger to speak with him one on one. Roger started screaming. When Rita asked what his problem was, Roger responded that he thought Kevin was going to smash his glasses into his face—just like his father had done.

The day before the scheduled time to return the boys, Rita and Kevin took them on a picnic. The boys both became agitated about returning to their father and asked to stay with their mother. Roger again defecated in his pants during this incident. Convinced that the boys were being abused by their father and afraid that he would show up and take the children, Rita came to the shelter. She was willing to let the children be taken to a foster home rather than have them return to Jack.

Rita did not know what to do. She thought she had joint custody but was told by Jack and his attorney that she had given up joint custody when she had left the children in Jack's care. She had no job, no family, and no financial support. Kevin was staying close to the shelter and living alone.

## *ASSESSMENT AND DIAGNOSTIC IMPRESSIONS*

### *Impressions and Assessment of Rita*

Assessment of victims of domestic violence requires a multimethod approach (O'Leary and Murphy, 1999). Principles of assessment include

1. data collection about multiple ecosystems;
2. data from the person, significant others, and direct observation of the client in the environment;
3. data on all critical variables about the person (cognitive, emotional, physical);
4. data about all parts of the children's lives (social functioning, emotional development); and

5. integration of the data into a comprehensive picture of the person and her environment (Allen-Meares and Lane, 1993).

In working with victims of domestic violence the foremost task is to establish the level of perpetrator lethality and to develop a safety plan (Davies, 1998). Perpetrators of domestic violence use psychological tactics to undermine their partners' self-confidence and autonomy. A woman leaving a relationship does not mean the assaults will stop. Rita's presence in the shelter and her determination to remain in the shelter until the safety of her and her children could be assured assisted in accomplishing this first task. As an advocate for her safety, the social worker would review with her the physical, psychological, financial, and child-related risks of remaining away from the perpetrator using the Battered Women's Analysis: Batter-Generated Risks developed by Greater Hartford Legal Assistance (Davies, 1998).

Victims of domestic violence most often are suffering from posttraumatic stress disorder (PTSD), a subclassification of anxiety disorder in the *Diagnostic and Statistical Manual of Mental Disorders* (DSM-IV) (American Psychiatric Association, 1994; Davies, 1998; O'Leary and Murphy, 1999; Saunders, 1999). Rita verbalized the spiral of violence (Tully, 1999) she experienced over the years with her husband as the abuse increased in frequency and severity. She continues to experience the physical and psychological abuse from the perpetrator. Her belief that the perpetrator has the FBI watching her is indicative of a victim's feelings of powerlessness and a perpetrator's characteristic of omniscient control over his victim.

The Beck's Depression Scale (Beck et al., 1961) and Index of Self-Esteem (Hudson, 1999) is useful in determining the extent of Rita's depression and low self-esteem and serves as a basis for providing evaluation of treatment. A single-system design is implemented using the frequency of meals and duration of sleep—indicators she has mentioned regarding her depression. The single-system design also serves as a means for evaluating progress in the intervention.

Rita's story has many gaps, such as Kevin's involvement with the family, the support system available to this couple, and the legal custody of the children. One goal of the assessment process is to clarify these issues. Further intensive interviewing assessment, as recommended by Davies (1998), provides an integrated, comprehensive basis of Rita and her environment upon which treatment can be established.

## Impressions and Assessment of Children

Increasingly the symptoms and manifestations of domestic violence on children are being recognized. These children are the "invisible victims" (Osofsky, 1995).

### Lauren

In terms of psychosocial development (Erikson, 1963), infants are forming trust with their caregivers, which requires the ability to predict their actions and depend upon them. Hopelessness, disorganization, and inappropriate differentiation of the infant's versus the caregiver's needs can result in the child developing mistrust, thus, hindering Lauren's psychosocial adjustment (Newman and Newman, 1995).

Symptoms of domestic violence have been found (through measures of the heart rate and galvanic skin response) to cause stress to the fetus, resulting in severe physiological distress after birth (Sudermann and Jaffee, 1999). These symptoms can be manifested through the child's prolonged crying, irritability, difficulty sleeping, as well as disruption in eating and play exploration, all resulting in failure to thrive. Although Lauren is only six months old and was not directly involved with the majority of the violence between Rita and Jack, she was affected by the stress and depression incurred by her mother during the final phases preceding Rita's admission to the shelter. A physical and close monitoring of Lauren's behaviors will assist in Lauren's assessment.

### Roger

Female victims of domestic violence often leave because of threats toward the children (Smith, O'Connor, and Berthelsen, 1996). Seemingly this was the case for Rita, especially in relation to Roger's behaviors.

Dozens of reports associating the witnessing of domestic violence and child development problems have been published. An estimated 11 to 20 percent of adults remember seeing, as children, violent incidences between their parental figures (Henning et al., 1996). Children observing violence in the home grow up confused about the meaning of love, violence, and intimacy (Wolak and Finkelhor, 1998).

The symptoms of this experience are widespread and long lasting, affecting every aspect of the child's life—both as a child and into the adult years:

1. behavioral aspects such as aggression, tantrums, immaturity, acting out, and delinquency;
2. emotional aspects such as anxiety, depression, low self-esteem, and depression;
3. physical aspects such as sleeplessness, eating disorders, and psychosomatic symptoms;
4. cognitive aspects such as poor academic performance; and
5. social aspects such as poor social skills and rejection by peers.

Signs of post-traumatic stress disorder include reexperiencing the event through nightmares, physical reactions such as headaches, shakiness, feeling numb, inability to remember important aspects of events, exaggerated startle response, and persistent, increased arousal (Wolak and Finkelhor, 1998).

Roger and his older brother Alfred are in Erikson's (1963) psychosocial developmental stage of industry versus inferiority. As a result of the violence in the home, Roger most likely was unable to achieve the earlier stages of psychosocial development and has regressed to earlier stages of development. His lack of self-worth and feelings of guilt are negatively affecting his biopsychosocial development. His severe regression and aggressive acts suggest that he is suffering from post-traumatic stress disorder. The Children's Impact of Traumatic Events Scale, Family Violence Version, measuring for trauma and its impact (Wolfe and Lehmann, 1992), or the Trauma Symptom Checklist for Children (Briere, 1996), measuring anxiety, depression, anger, under- and overarousal, dissociation, and sexual concerns, would assist in the assessment process.

## Alfred

Boys who witness domestic violence are at great risk at maturation of abusing their adult partners (Gleason, 1995). Although Alfred's overt behaviors are not as severe as his younger brother's, witnessing the violence against his mother has inevitably negatively impacted him and requires assessment and treatment. As he approaches adolescence, his behaviors may easily turn to hostility, aggression, running away, anxiety, and withdrawal (Sudermann and Jaffee, 1999).

During the interview process, building rapport and breaking the code of secrecy are major issues to address. Giving Alfred latitude in controlling the interview will assist in rapport building. Subtle symptoms, common to children witnessing domestic violence, need to be assessed, such as responses and attitudes about conflict resolution, assigning responsibility for violence, and knowledge and skills in dealing with violent incidents. Tools for assessment include the Child Behavior Checklist (Achenbach and Edelbrock, 1983), the Youth Self Report Form (Achenbach, 1991) of overall adjustment, or the Child Witness to Violence Interview (Jaffee, Wolfe, and Wilson, 1990).

## *Impressions and Assessment of the Family*

According to Weltner's family classification model (Paquin and Bushorn, 1993), Rita and her family would be considered to be at level one. Level one is indicative of a family at the lowest of the five levels of family functioning according to the types of problems with which they are struggling and the existing level of family organization. The family lacks leadership and struggles to meet the basic nurturance and protection needs of its members such as food, shelter, protection, clothing, and medical care.

In assessing this type of family the focus must be on its strengths. Various techniques for assessment include ecomaps diagramming the family's current connections with the environment including extended family and other social support systems, and genograms allowing condensing a large amount of information for identifying intrafamilial patterns over time (Paquin and Bushorn, 1993). More intense assessment procedures, such as the McMaster model of family functioning by Epstein, Bishop, and Baldwin, as noted in Paquin and Bushorn (1993), using six dimensions to categorize the structure, organization, and transactional patterns of family—problem solving, roles, communications, affective responsiveness, affective involvement, and behavior control—would be more appropriate after the family has achieved its basic needs.

## *Further Data-Gathering Techniques*

In addition to using scales and interviews to gather assessment data, other information is required to enable effective intervention. Intervention for the various members of the family would be initiated immediately; however, with the assistance of the case manager, additional information would be sought. This information includes

1. school records on the children;
2. medical examinations on Rita and all three children;
3. court records to determine the status of the children's custody; and
4. information from other agencies with which the family has had contact, such as the Division of Family Services.

## *IDENTIFICATION OF THE PROBLEM SOURCE AND MANIFESTATIONS*

### *Identified Problems*

Presenting problems by Rita were

1. stress,
2. Roger's emotional problems, and
3. custody of the children.

Social worker's identified problems were as follows:

1. Safety for Rita and children
2. PTSD of Rita
3. PTSD of Roger
4. Psychological problems of Alfred
5. Health care for children
6. Custody of children
7. Lack of basic needs for family (housing, food, clothing)
8. Lack of social support
9. Other health-related issues for the family (spirituality)

## INTERVENTION STRATEGIES AND SKILLS TO ELIMINATE BOTH THE SOURCES AND MANIFESTATIONS OF THE PROBLEMS

### Direct Intervention

Intervening with Rita requires remaining sensitive to how she is experiencing this situation and treating her as a unique individual (Davies, 1998). Listening skills are extremely important in developing a relationship between the social worker and Rita. That Rita is from a rural area also presents specific problems in obtaining safety and services (Fishwick, 1998).

The social worker needs to build Rita's confidence in her ability to overcome her problems. Supportive comments such as "You're handling so much" and "I admire your strength to cope with all you're dealing with" are important for her to hear and believe (Davies, 1998).

The social worker encourages Rita to discuss her spiritual beliefs and, if desired, to become involved with a local group—one in which she can still have safety from potential abuse. A battered woman may have deep spiritual beliefs and faith that provide her with additional strength and direction to face risks and implement plans (Davies, 1998).

Rita's participation in an educational group and a therapeutic group assists her in identifying with other women who have experienced domestic violence and in becoming empowered to free herself from oppression. Interaction with these women helps to establish a support system.

A goal of the social worker is to build a partnership or alliance with Rita. This therapy bonding can be assisted through agreement on established goals and on therapeutic tasks used to reach goals (O'Leary and Murphy, 1999). Goals include (1) becoming financially stable, (2) becoming emotionally healthy, and (3) developing a support system.

Due to the present unstable situation of the family, Roger will receive inpatient treatment for post-traumatic stress disorder at a local facility.

Alfred begins group treatment in the shelter with the goals of resolving the crisis he is experiencing, identifying and expressing his feelings, learning problem-solving skills, and learning healthy coping behaviors (Alessi and Hearn, 1998). Group counseling is the most widely suggested intervention for children from homes in which domestic violence has taken place (Ragg and Webb, 1992; Tutty and Wagar, 1994).

Family sessions conducted once a week include Kevin on occasion. Goals include establishing open communication among the family members, establishing Rita as the leader of her home (perhaps with the assistance of Kevin), and establishing healthy boundaries between family members.

To accomplish the goals established for the individual family members and the family as a whole, the social worker needs to be a mediator, advocate, broker, coordinator, and educator. These roles take place on the micro-, mezzo-, and macrolevels.

## *Indirect Intervention*

Numerous other systems need to be engaged to assist Rita and the children to achieve healthy lives both now and in the future.

- *Family court system:* The court advocate from the shelter and the volunteer attorney for the shelter can assist in the process of determining custody of the children. Many times the court system needs education as to the detrimental effects domestic violence has on the children. Although the safety of Rita and the children are the primary concerns, obtaining child support for Lauren is a secondary objective.
- *Health providers:* Rita and the children need ongoing health coverage. Application will be made for Medicare.
- *Division of family services:* For a period of time Rita is eligible to receive welfare financial assistance for the children. Protective services for children needs to be informed of the situation to assist in investigating the present status of the father's home and to offer recommendations to the courts regarding the future placement of the children.
- *Employment skills:* Rita needs encouragment to learn employment skills during the limited welfare period. Self-confidence can be gained from her developing the ability to support her family.

- *Support system:* Rita's mother, family members, and friends need assessment as to their ability and willingness to work with Rita and the children as they work toward independence. The plans for Rita and Kevin's relationship need to be pursued. Kevin needs to commit to the role he plays in the lives of Rita and the children.
- *Housing:* Rita may stay in the shelter at least until her safety is assured. Eventually, she will need to obtain her own housing by applying for government subsidized housing.
- *Law enforcement:* Rita, similar to many victims of abuse, has a negative impression of law enforcement in the role of protection. Officers will be invited to speak to the women's group in an effort to teach self-protection and protection of the home as well as to reduce the negative stigma that can exist between victims of abuse and law enforcement. On a macrolevel basis, the social worker can take the role of educator with the law enforcement agencies to sensitize them to the problems and perceptions of victims of domestic violence.
- *Coalition building:* For Rita, as well as the many other families experiencing domestic violence, the social worker facilitates the development of a coalition with the mission of eradicating family violence. Members of the coalition would include representatives from the court system, emergency services, schools, universities, criminal justice system, government agencies, law enforcement, and numerous other private companies and public agencies.

## *STRATEGIES TO EVALUATE INTERVENTION*

Evaluating the outcome of intervention is essential to any professional. The social worker has established the means to evaluate an intervention by the baseline of single-system designs, the pretest scores on scales, and the establishing of objectives.

For the single-system design, the difference between the client's behaviors before intervention and after intervention can be determined by using the points on the celeration line. The determination of a significant difference can be established merely by eyeballing the line or by calculating the difference using the appropriate statistical procedure.

The scales for determining Rita's level of depression and self-esteem would be readministered to determine the difference before and after intervention. The scales used for the children would also be readministered to determine the degree of change.

Each of the objectives on the treatment plan is evaluated to determine the level of achievement.

## *CONCLUSION*

The family health perspective requires social workers to assess and intervene with families using a wide variety of skills. Rita's case is typical of families experiencing domestic violence. Each family member needs to be considered as an individual and as part of the whole family system. Careful attention to detail is required encompassing the interaction between the family and its environment. Although demanding of resources, the family health perspective provides the most promising assessment and intervention process for empowering families to reach levels of maximum functioning for themselves and for society.

## REFERENCES

Achenbach, T. M. (1991). *Youth self report.* Burlington, VT: University Associates in Psychiatry.

Achenbach, T. M. and Edelbrock, C. S. (1983). *Manual for the child behavior checklist and revised child behavior profile.* Burlington, VT: University Associates in Psychiatry.

Alessi, J. J. and Hearn, K. (1998). Group treatment of children in shelters for battered women. In A. R. Roberts (Ed.), *Battered women and their families,* Second edition. (pp. 3-38). New York: Springer.

Allen-Meares, P. and Lane, B. A. (1993). Grounding social work practice in theory: Ecosystems. In J. B. Rauch (Ed.), *Assessment: A sourcebook for social work practice* (pp. 3-14). Milwaukee, WI: Families International.

American Psychiatric Association (1994). *Diagnostic and statistical manual of mental disorders,* Fourth edtion. Washington, DC; Author.

Beck, A. T., Ward, C. H., Mendelson, M., Mock, J., and Erbaugh, J. (1961). An inventory for measuring depression. *Archives of General Psychiatry, 5,* 53-63.

Briere, J. (1996). *Trauma symptom checklist for children.* San Antonio, TX: The Psychological Corporation/Harcourt Brace.

Davies, J. (1998). *Safety planning with battered women: Complex lives/difficult choices*. Thousand Oaks, CA: Sage.

Erikson, E. H. (1963). *Childhood and society,* Second edition. New York: Norton.

Fishwick, N. (1998). Issues in providing care for rural battered women. In J. C. Campbell (Ed.), *Empowering survivors of abuse: Health care for battered women and their children* (pp. 280-290). Thousand Oaks, CA: Sage.

Gleason, W. J. (1995). Children of battered women: Developmental delays and behavioral dysfunction. *Violence and Victims, 10* (2), 153-158.

Henning, K., Leitenberg, H., Coffey, P., Turner, T., and Bennett, R. T. (1996). Long-term psychological and social impact of witnessing physical conflict between parents. *Journal of Interpersonal Violence, 11*(1), 35-51.

Hudson, W. W. (1999). Index of Self-Esteem. In W. W. Hudson (Ed.), *WALMYR assessment scales scoring manual* (pp. 19, 52). Tallahassee, FL: WALMYR.

Jaffee, P. G., Wolfe, D.A., and Wilson, S. (1990). *Children of battered women*. Newbury Park, CA: Sage.

Newman, B. M. and Newman, P. R. (1995). *Development through life: A psychosocial approach,* Sixth edition. Pacific Groves, CA: Brooks/Cole Publishing.

O'Leary, K. D. and Murphy, C. (1999). Clinical issues in the assessment of partner violence. In R. T. Ammerman and M. Hersen (Eds.), *Assessment of family violence: A clinical and legal sourcebook,* Second edition (pp. 24-47). New York: John Wiley and Sons.

Osofsky, J. D. (1995). Children who witness domestic violence: The invisible victims. *Society for Research in Child Development, IX* (3), 1-20.

Paquin, G.W. and Bushorn, R.J. (1993). Family treatment assessment for novices. In J. B. Rauch (Ed.), *Assessment: A sourcebook for social work practice* (pp. 47-58). Milwaukee, WI: Families International.

Pardeck, J. T. and Yuen, F. K. (1997). A family health approach to social work practice. *Family Therapy, 24* (2), 115-128.

Ragg, D.M. and Webb, C. (1992). Group treatment for the preschool child witness of spouse abuse. *Journal of Child and Youth Care,* 7(1), 1-19.

Saunders, D. G. (1999).Woman battering. In R. T. Ammerman and M. Hersen (Eds.), *Assessment of family violence: A clinical and legal sourcebook,* Second edition (pp. 243-270). New York: John Wiley and Sons.

Smith, J., O'Connor, and Berthelsen, D. (1996). The effects of witnessing domestic violence on young children's psycho-social adjustment. *Australian Social Work, 49* (4), 3-10.

Sudermann, M. and Jaffee, P. G. (1999). Child witnesses of domestic violence. In R.T. Ammerman and M. Hersen (Eds.), *Assessment of family violence: A clinical and legal sourcebook,* Second edition (pp. 343-366). New York: John Wiley and Sons.

Tully, C. T. (1999). Hate crimes, domestic violence, and the lesbian and gay community. In J. C. McClennen and J. Gunther (Eds.), *A professional guide to under-*

*standing gay and lesbian domestic violence: Understanding practice interventions* (pp. 13-28). Lewiston, NY: The Edwin Mellen Press.

Tutty, L.M. and Wagar, J. (1994). The evolution of a group for young children who have witnessed family violence. *Social Work with Groups, 17* (1/2), 89-103.

Wolak, J. and Finkelhor, D. (1998). Effects of partner violence on children. In *Partner violence: A 20-year literature review and synthesis.* NNFR: Department of the Air Force. Accessed June 25. <http://www.nnfr.org/nnfr/research/pv_ch4.html>.

Wolfe, V. V. and Lehmann, P. J. (1992). The Children's Impact of Traumatic Events Scale—Family Violence Version. Unpublished assessment instrument. London, ON: Children's Hospital of Western Ontario.

Chapter 6

# Mental Health and Family Health Social Work Practice

Catherine L. Hawkins
Lisa Langston

In this chapter, a social worker in an outpatient behavioral health facility in a midsized town in the Midwest receives a referral for on-going treatment following a psychiatric hospitalization for a patient named Mary. During her five-day hospitalization, she was given a diagnosis of "Bipolar I Disorder, Most Recent Episode Manic, Severe, with Mood-Incongruent Psychotic Features." At discharge, the symptoms had decreased significantly and, according to hospital records, Mary indicated that she understood the importance of continuing with her lithium prescription. The following information was obtained during the assessment session that included Mary and her husband Ted.

## *ASSESSMENT AND DIAGNOSTIC IMPRESSION*

### *Social History*

Mary is a forty-four-year-old married female. She currently lives with her husband, Ted, age forty-six, and two of their three children, Brian, age fifteen, and Amanda, age nine. Their oldest child, Jenny, is twenty-three years old and lives in California. Mary's career has focused on writing; she currently runs her own freelance business in which she does both creative and technical writing. Ted works as a managing member of an architectural firm.

Mary is British and was raised in India until the age of fourteen when she was sent to boarding school in England. Ted was raised in St. Louis, Missouri, and met Mary (then age nineteen) when he was in London for his junior year abroad. The two married one year later and set up residence in St. Louis. Both report that soon after the birth of their first child at age twenty-one, Mary began to experience periods of decreased activity and low mood, alternating with periods of increased activity and inflated mood. Mary was comfortable with these moods and learned to use them to boost her creativity and productivity as a writer.

When she was thirty, Mary and Ted adopted an infant son from India. At age thirty-two she experienced her first true manic episode, sought psychiatric treatment, and was prescribed lithium. Although this medication effectively leveled her mood, she also felt that it "took away [her] creative edge," and she stopped taking it after three months. She appeared to return to her previous pattern of milder mood swings and managed without medication for a number of years.

The couple adopted a second infant from India, a girl, when Mary was thirty-six. At thirty-seven, Mary experienced a second manic episode which this time also included paranoid beliefs. She saw a psychiatrist once again, began taking lithium again, and within days experienced lucid thinking and a level mood. Mary continued her prescribed lithium treatment for fourteen months. During subsequent years, Mary periodically used lithium when she became symptomatic. With each episode, her symptoms increased in severity.

The episode that precipitated this most recent hospitalization came when Ted had been out of town for a month on a business trip to Europe. Mary had become increasingly agitated and fearful following his departure, and over the course of the four weeks slept less and was more active. Due to a growing fear that one of their cars might break down, Mary purchased two new vehicles. As only one car fit in the garage, she left the other on the street. Fearful that someone would steal it, she decided to mar its appearance so that it would be less desirable to a thief. With a hammer she severely damaged the outside and inside of the vehicle. A witnessing neighbor phoned the police. They took Mary to a hospital emergency room.

Both Brian and Amanda had become increasingly concerned about their mother over the four weeks that their father was gone. Initially, Brian began to feel angry that his mother was "getting all weird" again, while Amanda tried to help her mother feel better and keep things together. During the hammer attack, Brian left and went to a friend's home. Amanda stayed, begging her mother not to do anything with the hammer, and called her paternal aunt for help.

Ted learned about Mary's episode and hospitalization from his sister who called him in Europe. He was concerned about Mary and immediately made plans to return to St. Louis. Upon returning, he visited Mary and then told the children their mother would be home soon but did not address any of their feelings regarding the incident or their mother's behavior. His goal was to organize the house and help provide a stable environment for the children.

## *Assessment of Parents*

Marital discord was obvious from the first meeting with Mary and Ted. Ted was angry with Mary for "having messed things up again" and for not having trusted him enough to tell him about her fears of being harmed. He believed that she could control her actions if she chose to and that he might have been able to prevent the recent incident from happening if she had confided in him. Mary continues to mistrust Ted and is hurt that he holds her responsible for actions over which she believes she had no control. They note significant differences in their overall styles. Mary is open, creative, spontaneous, and requires minimal organization. Ted is structured, organized, and extremely consistent in his habits and preferences. Mary tends to lose track of time and fails to follow through on family and household tasks, while Ted tracks daily routines and events carefully, becoming upset if small details are missed. Their parenting styles reflect their personality styles. Mary is involved with and attentive to the children's emotional and creative needs but frequently forgets their schedules and details regarding their lives. Ted ensures that they make it to all their activities but is more distant emotionally. With the arrival of each child and the progression of Mary's symptoms, Mary and Ted have become increasingly polarized in their styles. This polarization is not a problem when all is going smoothly with the family, and they find ways to work around their differences. Their love for each other is clear, but when crises arise they experience marital and parental difficulties. Each resents the other's operating style.

## Assessment of Children

Amanda, age nine, exhibits characteristics of a parentified child. She has assumed this role to maintain family functioning. Amanda has assumed her mother's functions to protect her mother. It is now part of who she is. Developmentally, Amanda is in the stage of middle childhood. According to Newman and Newman (1995), middle childhood is characterized by the importance of parent/child relationships, peer friendships, and participation in meaningful interpersonal communication. Successful transitions through these stages would help prepare Amanda for adolescence, but because she has assumed some adult roles, her peer friendships and participation in age-appropriate social activity have suffered. At this age, Amanda still needs the comfort of family members and should be exploring more complex social relationships with peers and other significant adults. Cultural issues are also important. Amanda looks different from her parents and her friends have commented about those differences. This may be a significant reason that Amanda assumed an important role within the family and has not ventured out into her social community.

Brian (age fifteen) is moving through the developmental stage of early adolescence. Newman and Newman (1995) describe normal negative adolescent emotions as embarrassment, anxiety, shame, guilt, and anger. Even if Brian's family were functioning at an optimal level, he still might experience the anger he has exhibited. With the family dysfunction, Brian is experiencing intensified feelings of embarrassment, shame, guilt, and anger. In addition, Brian is undergoing physical changes typical to adolescence. He is attempting to distance himself from his family. Overall, Brian is at greater risk for problems such as depression and acting out to minimize the embarrassment and shame of his mother's behavior. Culturally, Brian is also of Indian descent. Although he has often wondered about his cultural heritage, he has not yet begun to explore what this means to him. His peer group has readily accepted him.

The twenty-three-year-old biological daughter, Jenny, is a somewhat unknown factor within the family. She left the family when she was eighteen and put great geographical distance between herself and family. Jenny also experienced her mother's erratic behavior (albeit at a less dramatic stage). She may be concerned about inheriting her mother's illness. She has visited the family only twice since moving to California. Jenny did express to her mother during her last visit that she was thinking about seeking some counseling for herself.

## *Family Strengths*

This family functions well when undue stress is not a factor. Evidence of good communication between and among the family members exists and they have been successful, at times, in meeting one another's needs. Each member has the capacity to further the family's development to a higher state of holistic well-being. Intelligence and education are major assets of each member of this family. They are capable of at least intellectually understanding the biological, psychological, social, emotional, and spiritual problems occurring within the family. Resourcefulness is another strength. Because they are financially comfortable and able to attain resources outside the family system, achieving a higher state of holistic well-being is possible. In addition, Mary has responded to treatment for bipolar disorder in the past, indicating a good prognosis for her and the entire family. These combined strengths place this family at an advantage over those with fewer resources. Further, good insurance coverage is helpful; a lack of adequate insurance coverage for behavioral health issues is a major policy issue for disenfranchised families.

## *SOURCE OF THE PROBLEM AND MANIFESTATIONS*

1. Mary's medication management (SOURCE)
2. Enhancing family's knowledge of mental illness (MANIFESTATION)
3. Enhancing the children's psychological and emotional well-being (as a function of medication management—MANIFESTATION; as a function of adoption—SOURCE)
4. Parenting skills (SOURCE)
5. Cultural and spiritual issues for Amanda and Brian (SOURCE)

## *INTERVENTION STRATEGIES AND SKILLS*

Ongoing sessions will be scheduled with Mary and her family on a weekly basis, and the following interventions will be made.

1. Due to the chronic nature of bipolar disorder and Mary's need for medication, she was encouraged to continue taking her prescription upon discharge from the hospital. When she did not, the social worker made a referral to a psychiatrist and verified that Mary kept the appointment. Support for regimen compliance was a necessary part of the intervention. Due to Mary's tendency to stop taking medication once she feels stable, the following contingency plans were made. She was encouraged to monitor her own thought processes and share her doubts about prescription compliance. She was also encouraged to share any thoughts of stopping the medication with Ted, the psychiatrist, and this social worker. As Mary's believes the medication curtails her creative edge, she was warned to consider carefully the negative consequences of discontinuing her prescription and encouraged to find ways to further her creative processes while taking the medication. Ted, Brian, and Amanda talked to Mary about their experiences when she stops taking her medication. The children involved Ted in these discussions. The social worker was available to aid Mary throughout.

2. Because Mary and her family had received no education about bipolar disorder, the social worker, in conjunction with other mental health professionals, provided this information. Information regarding the disorder's nature, course, symptoms, and the need for ongoing medication were addressed. In addition, information on the impact of mental illness on family relationships was given. All family members' questions were addressed, and the need for mutual and outside support was stressed. Referrals were made to a local support group for individuals with mental illness and their families. The genogram was used to increase awareness of historical patterns of behavior and roles adopted by members of the extended family. All family members considered the probable consequences of continuing these historical patterns.

3. Given Brian's age and current developmental stage (adolescence), distancing himself some from the family was expected. The ways in which he did so, and the intense anger surrounding his actions, however, were troubling. The parents were educated about the

appropriateness of the developmental tasks in adolescence. The parents were also taught about Brian's anger and appropriate responses. Family interventions targeted the need for increased autonomy and constructive responses to crises. Brian rated his anger daily on a 1 to 10 scale (with 10 being most angry). On the days in which it reached at least 6, he was expected to talk to the parent toward whom he was experiencing anger. The family was educated about Amanda's parentified child role. The negative long- and short-term impacts were explained including the special impact this role has on the development tasks during latency. Interventions encouraged Amanda to step away from the role to develop friendships and activities with her peers. To this end, both parents monitored Amanda's behavior daily and noted any parental functions. If caught, Amanda was stopped and the parents performed the function themselves. They also monitored Amanda's emotional responses to these interventions. She usually felt relieved, although occasionally she felt sad and anxious as this role made her feel special and important. In addition, Mary planned activities in which she clearly was in the role of mother and Amanda in the role of daughter. Finally, the rift between Jenny and her parents was addressed in family therapy. Mary and Ted attempted to contact Jenny to rebuild their relationship with her. Initial overtures were unsuccessful. Brian and Amanda also needed some support and information regarding their adoptions. Both parents provided the information, and external support group attendance (as needed) was encouraged.

4. Standard supportive treatment was used to resolve the hurt and anger Mary and Ted felt toward one another and to address the polarization of parental roles. Each parent was provided parent skills training based on the local county's department of family resources training model. Each parent examined his or her role and the degree to which he or she was entrenched in these patterns of behavior. Subsequent interventions focused on increasing Ted's emotional awareness and involvement, and at helping Mary to develop organizational and time management skills. Ted noted each family member's apparent emotional state at least one time each day and observed Mary's responses to emotional concerns. Mary purchased a calendar and wrote down family events and observed Ted and the methods he used to remember their schedules. Without changing their personalities, the increased awareness of their different operating styles improved both

parents' adaptability and tolerance. New skills enhanced their parenting abilities.

5. The final concerns related to cultural and spiritual issues. Even though the two younger children were born in India, little had been done to educate them regarding their cultural and spiritual heritage. Because Mary was raised in India, she led efforts to explore these two areas. She shared information from her own experience with Indian customs and Buddhist philosophy. The children researched areas of interest and were given opportunities to meet (in person, through e-mail, or letters) other children their age of Indian descent. Both parents helped, as appropriate. In addition, this provided an opportunity for Ted to learn more about Mary's heritage and historical experience.

As the family began to stabilize, sessions were scheduled less frequently (e.g. every other week, then monthly). Due to the chronic nature of Mary's illness, however, the social worker was available to the family on an as-needed basis following the end of formal treatment. Eventually, regular yet infrequent appointments (every eight to twelve weeks) were maintained. The purpose was to continuously assess the status of Mary's symptoms, determine her compliance with recommended medical intervention, and insure that positive changes in family dynamics were maintained.

## *STRATEGIES TO EVALUATE INTERVENTION*

1. Each day, Ted checked his wife's pillbox to see if she was complying with her medication regimen. Conceivably, Mary could have thrown out her pills to make Ted think she had taken them. However, Ted monitored her behavior in concert with her medication routine. Ted did not notice any inconsistent behaviors. Apparently, Mary was more compliant (and honest) with her doctor's recommendations when monitored. Further, Mary marked on her calendar the days in which she had self-doubts about taking her medication. Over the six-month period of intervention, Mary had four days of self-doubt. Following discussions with the social worker and her husband, Mary was more likely to agree with her psychiatrist about the importance of continuing her medication.

2. Attendance at support groups by family members was tallied. Information and emotional impressions were shared between family members and the social worker.

3. Whenever Brian had angry outbursts, he would self-rate the outburst on a scale of 1 to 10 (with ten being most angry). He would then report his anger and its rating to the precipitating family member to discuss the issue. Brian's number of outbursts decreased from about one to two per day to about one per week by the end of treatment. The parents also monitored Amanda's behavior, charting her emotional responses on a 1 to 10 scale. As the number of role-clarifying behaviors by Mary increased, Amanda's behaviors improved. Finally, calls to Jenny were counted. In the six-month period, Jenny was called at least weekly with six personal contacts and nineteen answering machine messages. Jenny never returned calls after receiving messages. Personal contact by phone was met with minimal enthusiasm by Jenny. Attendance at adoption support groups was tallied for each child. Information and emotional impressions were shared between family members and the social worker.

4. Subsequent interventions focused on increasing Ted's emotional awareness and involvement and helping Mary to develop organizational and time management skills.

5. "Classes" on Indian culture were held each Thursday night from 6:30 to 8:00 p.m. each week by Mary in the home. The sessions were never missed and each week, both children (except for a three-week session in which Brian was having a difficult time emotionally) were able to make new friends. All information collected by the children was shared with the family.

Various self-reports by each family member were used. The two younger children kept weekly journals regarding their own feelings, perceptions, and a plan of action for troubling situations. They evaluated their perception of each of the other family members with regard to effectiveness of communication, degree of success with outside support, and comfort level in handling stressful family situations.

## REFERENCE

Newman, B.M. and Newman, P.R. (1995). *Development through life: A psychosocial approach,* Sixth edition. Pacific Grove, CA: Brooks/Cole Publishing Company.

# Chapter 7

# Family Health Practice in a Medical Setting with an Infant and Her Family

Melissa A. Hollis
Gregory J. Skibinski

In hearing the term *family health,* people might think of how medical problems affect families. Family health, of course, is more than that. In this chapter the authors present a medical case of an infant and how the illness affected her family.

Working with families with a newborn in an intensive care nursery (ICN) can be a very interesting and challenging experience. This chapter discusses a social worker's interactions with an ICN family using the family health perspective. The authors present a social history of the family including a diagnostic impression, followed by source and manifestation information, intervention strategies, and intervention evaluation methods. A discussion of different levels of practice is included, along with pertinent family health skills, and the theory base used in this case.

## *ASSESSMENT AND DIAGNOSTIC IMPRESSIONS*

### Social History

*Background Information Obtained Prior to First Meeting*

Theresa and Don are an unmarried, Caucasian couple living in a midsized Midwestern town. They were referred to hospital social services after the premature birth of their daughter, Stacy, and her subsequent admission to the intensive care nursery. Theresa is twenty-one years old and her boyfriend Don is twenty-six. Theresa has never been married. Don was married to another woman for about one year and has been divorced from her for the past two years; the marriage produced no children. Stacy is the first child of Theresa and Don. Theresa is currently unemployed. Following a period of unemployment, Don has recently returned to work with a local company. Theresa infrequently attends a local Methodist church with her parents. No known previous social work intervention has occurred.

## *Presenting Problem*

The primary presenting problem, and in this case crisis, is that Stacy was born prematurely (at thirty weeks gestation), causing life-threatening physical problems requiring admission to the ICN and extensive home care upon discharge. The premature birth has caused breathing difficulties (apnea—the secession of breathing), eating difficulties due to an immature digestive system, and poor sucking response. Stacy is currently on an apnea monitor, tube feedings, and receives eating training from a speech therapist. Growth and developmental problems are common for such children.

All other information was obtained from family interviews, observations, and multidisciplinary discussions.

## **Social Worker Assessment**

### *Family Relationships*

Theresa and Don reported no difficulties in their relationship. They dated about six months before the pregnancy. They lived together intermittently during the pregnancy. At times Theresa lived with her parents, and at other times Theresa and Don lived together with friends. They spent some nights in Don's car.

Theresa's parents adopted her as an infant; she has no contact with her biological parents. Her adoptive parents visited Stacy often and Theresa reports they are supportive. Stress in the parent/daughter relationship occurs because Theresa's parents do not believe a couple should live together without being married. Her parents will not let Don stay in their home with Theresa. Also, Theresa's parents have given her a two-month deadline to "do something with your life or move out of this house."

Don's parents are supportive financially and emotionally. They live in a small town outside the city, making a few trips to the city hospital where Stacy is receiving care.

Little is known of Theresa's relationship with her adoptive siblings. They are many years older than Theresa and were living on their own by the time she was about seven years old. Theresa has had no contact with her five biological siblings, all of whom were already in foster care when Theresa was adopted. Her two adoptive sisters live in another state and did not visit Stacy during her hospitalization. Don has one brother, who lives in his hometown twenty-four miles away. Don did not discuss his brother during Stacy's hospital stay, and his brother did not visit the hospital.

*Communication Patterns*

Verbal communication patterns among Theresa and Don and the hospital staff varied. At times Theresa and Don were able to give and receive information clearly; at other times, staff heard them yelling, and the couple sometimes used profanity with nursery staff. An example of such communication occurred when a nurse asked Theresa not to use profanity at Stacy's bedside or she would have to leave the nursery. Theresa then swore at the nurse. Later that night, Theresa was able to discuss the situation with the nurse and claimed she understood why it is wrong to use profanity in the nursery.

Theresa also ignored nursing staff requests to comply with some hospital protocols. In one such case, a nurse asked Theresa to remove her hand from the oxygen portal of Stacy's isolette. The nurse explained that Theresa could use the other portal to touch Stacy. Theresa did not speak to the nurse or remove her hand from the portal, thus obstructing the proper flow of oxygen. Don reportedly did not support the nurse's request. Theresa and Don left shortly after the incident, at which time Stacy had to be placed under an oxygen hood because of her increased oxygen needs.

Theresa also repeatedly missed training sessions in the use of an apnea monitor. When nursing staff and the social worker later questioned her, Theresa reported she was not going to do something that was not needed. Staff informed both Theresa and Don that the training was required to take Stacy home, but both refused to complete the training. Based on this refusal and previous behaviors, staff made a hotline call to the Division of Family Services (DFS). In response to the call that day, the DFS caseworker came to see the family at the hospital and explained that she was the assigned social worker. After the DFS worker left, Theresa and Don got into a fight in the nursery. Theresa ripped up the DFS worker's business card, yelled at Don, and hit him before storming out of the nursery.

Their nonverbal communication also varied. Staff often observed the two being gentle with Stacy and with each other. At other times, they gave each other and hospital staff antagonistic looks, and on one occasion Theresa slapped Don while they were in the nursery.

Difficulties surfaced again when Theresa became hostile with the speech therapist who was teaching Stacy to eat. Theresa refused to let her demonstrate feeding techniques and did not respond to questions or opportunities to practice. Theresa reportedly stated that Stacy would eat when she was ready and did not want anyone to help her. The therapist attempted to explain the purpose of the training, but Theresa became increasingly hostile and refused further interaction.

*Behavioral Patterns*

Theresa and Don exhibited poor problem-solving skills; the social worker observed these difficulties, and ICN staff reported them as well. Theresa's typical behavior was to flee a difficult situation, then act as if the problems never existed or that her flight never occurred. Don often reacted by pursuing her. He, too, rarely acknowledged that anything had happened. For example, Theresa walked away from a physician who was explaining the medical necessity of a blood transfusion for Stacy. Another example occurred when Theresa and Don were to start training in the use of a home apnea monitor. Theresa announced she had to go to the restroom and never returned. Don attempted to find her, but neither of them returned for the training that day.

*Occupational Situation*

Theresa and Don met while working for the same local company, where Don still works. Neither was employed when Stacy was born, but Don did return to his inventory job during her hospitalization. Don likes the flexible hours, although he finds the work tedious. His hourly rate is just above minimum wage.

## Physical Health of Family Members

Theresa and Don have no reported physical health problems. Stacy's only health problems are the result of her premature birth. She was eventually sent home from the hospital on medications and with a home apnea monitor. She required tube feedings to supplement her oral intake. The degree of long-term effects of prematurity is presently unclear, and a developmental evaluation was scheduled at six months of age.

## Involvement of Community Institutions

Theresa gains some support from her church attendance. Her pastor visited with the family throughout Stacy's hospital stay. Theresa's parents report she had learning problems in school, saying she could handle only one subject at a time. She dropped out of high school following tenth grade and does not have a GED. Don graduated from high school and is taking courses at the local technical college. He took a leave of absence from school while Stacy was hospitalized. Neither Theresa or Don are involved in any clubs or other community activities.

## Client-Identified Problems

Aside from the medical needs of their daughter, Theresa and Don also identified financial concerns as a problem. They requested assistance for food and gasoline expenses as well as financial help in establishing their own household. They had difficulty asking for such assistance, even though it was necessary for Stacy's hospital discharge.

## **Summary**

The crisis of having a premature child and the child's subsequent ICN hospitalization were difficult for this family. The stress of the situation brought forth the less desirable characteristics of the family, and they demonstrated limited coping mechanisms and only moderate social support. This was evidenced by Theresa's use of profanity toward hospital staff and her pattern of ignoring and fleeing difficult situations.

As a couple, Theresa and Don tried to present themselves as functioning well, yet problems became more evident as time passed. It seemed they desired to be good parents but had not learned effective communication or parenting skills. The following information serves as a summary of this case.

## PROBLEM SOURCES AND MANIFESTATIONS

A. Presenting problems
  1. Medical problems due to premature birth (SOURCE)
     a. Breathing difficulties
     b. Eating difficulties
  2. Potential developmental difficulties (SOURCE)
B. Client-identified problem
  1. Stress (generalized) but especially financial (MANIFESTATION)
C. Social worker–identified problems
  1. Deficit of illness-specific child care skills (MANIFESTATION)
  2. Limited coping skills (SOURCE)
     a. Poor verbal communication
     b. Volatile temper
     c. Withdrawal from stressful situations
  3. Moderate social support (SOURCE)

## INTERVENTION STRATEGIES AND ACTIVITIES TO ELIMINATE BOTH SOURCES AND MANIFESTATIONS

In this case, the assessment, planning, intervention, and evaluation processes were very intertwined and developmental in nature. Working with this family required a multidisciplinary approach. Input from nursing staff, physicians, therapists, and other social workers proved beneficial to understanding the family's situation and Stacy's medical needs.

Work with this family focused on evaluating the family's functioning and the parents' ability to meet Stacy's care needs. As concerns began to surface about the couple's abilities, a plan was needed to address those needs. A family conference was scheduled, allowing social services and nursing staff to discuss the situation with Theresa and Don. The nurse explained Stacy's medical condition and treatment. She also provided an opportunity for Theresa and Don to ask questions.

Following the conference, the social worker met with Theresa and Don in an attempt to understand the cause of their difficulties. Neither was willing to discuss any underlying issues or concerns. They acknowledged they were stressed but requested only financial assistance to establish a home for their new family. They were having difficulty finding housing in their price range through newspaper want ads. They agreed to compile a budget to see what they would be able to afford and to explore any possible financial assistance from their families. The social worker looked into community resources.

After the conference, intervention focused on living quarters and Stacy's needs following discharge. The couple found accomodations to rent and obtained funds from community agencies to pay the first month's rent, which freed Theresa and Don's money to pay the utility deposit and start phone service. They used a crib stored at Don's parents house and reported that they had clothing, bottles, diapers, and other necessities.

The DFS worker arranged to meet with Theresa and Don a few days after the conference. The social worker met with the DFS caseworker before that meeting to discuss the case and to obtain a release of information so medical information from Stacy's hospital chart could be shared with the DFS worker before meeting with Theresa and Don. Theresa, Don, and Theresa's pastor were in the ICN waiting room, where Don and the pastor were trying to talk Theresa into meeting with the DFS worker.

The DFS worker and the social worker spoke with Don and the pastor. They explained that a social worker is a mandated reporter of child endangerment and that Stacy has medical care needs. The DFS worker explained that she has to meet with Stacy's parents before any decisions are made and that if both parents were not willing to meet with her, she would have to take action on behalf of Stacy. Don and the pastor again went to talk with Theresa in the waiting room. Staff saw Theresa come out of the waiting room, push Don out of her way, and exit the nursery area. The DFS worker did meet with Don and the pastor on that day and with Theresa at a later date.

Due to Stacy's multiple medical needs, those involved considered a medical foster care placement. After meeting with the family and evaluating the home, the DFS social worker, in conjunction with the juvenile office worker, decided that Theresa and Don could try to take Stacy home. DFS did assign a caseworker to follow the family at home. Once that decision was made, intervention plans were quickly developed because Stacy was almost ready for discharge.

Nursing staff continued to educate Theresa and Don on Stacy's needs. The couple attended CPR (cardiopulmonary resuscitation) classes and apnea monitor training. Staff set up some health care nursing visits and speech therapy. The social worker arranged for the family's enrollment in the Parents As Teachers and First Steps programs to ensure continued education, support, and monitoring. She helped Theresa and Don complete the necessary forms for the Women, Infants, and Children (WIC) nutrition program. At three months of age, hospital staff sent Stacy home with her parents.

The following is a summary of the activities involved in this case:

1. Medical problems due to premature birth (SOURCE)
   a. Breathing difficulties: apnea monitor training as needed. Competency established by one parent prior to discharge.
   b. Eating difficulties: tube feeding training as needed. Competency established by one parent prior to discharge.
2. Potential developmental difficulties (SOURCE)
   a. Community resources
   b. Parents As Teachers program
   c. First Steps program
   d. WIC program
   e. Premature baby support group
   f. Developmental examination at six months of age
3. Stress (generalized) but especially financial (MANIFESTATION)
   a. Stress inoculation training
   b. Prepare budget
   c. Financial assistance
   d. Set up house-hunting strategy

4. Deficit of illness-specific child care skills (MANIFESTATION)
   a. Apnea monitoring
   b. Tube feedings
   c. CPR training
   d. Home health care nursing home visits (both a source of parental skill development and child care monitor)
5. Limited coping skills (SOURCE)
   a. Communication skills training
   b. Community resources: Parents As Teachers, First Steps, WIC
6. Moderate social support (SOURCE)
   a. Recruit grandparents to provide some economic support, social and parenting tasks, and visits (e.g., providing the crib)
   b. Community resources: Parents As Teachers, First Steps, WIC

## *STRATEGIES TO EVALUATE INTERVENTION*

### *Evaluation by Medical Professionals*

The medical professionals provided the parents with training for the child's medical needs (apnea, tube feedings, and CPR training). The parents completed all training prior to discharge. Parental competence was based on professional judgment.

Medical and developmental examinations by a physician were scheduled three months after discharge. A registered nurse visited the home weekly to monitor the progress of the child and family. The nurse also monitored the quality of the tube feedings and the family's compliance with the WIC program. The measures of compliance were be determined by the child's growth and development. The social workers administering the WIC program monitored compliance based on parental activities.

### *Evaluation by Social Worker*

Parental competence was to be monitored by social workers involved in the Parents As Teachers and the First Steps programs. The parents completed the program with minimal competence based on the professional judgment of the social worker. The social workers also evaluated their communication skills. Propriety of the home environment was evaluated by DFS using modifications to the Family

Risk Scales (Magura and Moses, 1987) and the Child Well-Being Scales (Magura, Moses, and Jones, 1987). The parents also completed a stress-inoculation training course. Success was determined by completion of the course, attendance, and role-play performance. Following course completion, the parents were each asked to complete the Index of Clinical Stress (Hudson and Abell, 1992) and the Index of Self-Esteem (Hudson, 1993). Finally, the family's amount of social support was measured by the Provision of Social Relations scale (Turner, Frankel, and Levin, 1983).

## *EPILOGUE*

Despite such extensive intervention, Stacy was readmitted to the hospital for failure to thrive a few weeks after leaving the nursery. Fortunately, the intervention plan included various professionals who quickly identified lapses in Stacy's progress. Stacy was later discharged from the hospital to the primary care of her maternal grandmother. Similar intervention plans and programs were implemented to assist the grandmother in her duties. The child is currently doing well.

## REFERENCES

Hudson, W. W. (1993). Index of Self-Esteem. In Nugent, W. R., Sieppert, J. D., and Hudson, W. W. (2001). *Practice Evaluation for the 21st Century* (p. 412). Belmont, CA: Brooks/Cole.

Hudson, W. W. and Abell, N. (1992). Index of Clinical Stress. In Nugent, W. R., Sieppert, J. D., and Hudson, W. W. (2001). *Practice Evaluation for the 21st Century* (p. 408). Belmont, CA: Brooks/Cole.

Magura, S. and Moses, B. S. (1987). *Outcome Measures for Child Welfare Services: Child Well-Being Scales and Rating Form.* Washington, DC: Child Welfare League of America.

Magura, S., Moses, B. S., and Jones, M. A. (1987). *Assessing Risk and Measuring Change in Families: The Family Risk Scales.* Washington, DC: Child Welfare League of America.

Turner, R. J., Frankel, B. G., and Levin, D. M. (1983). Social support: Conceptualization, measurement, and implications for mental health. *Research in Community and Mental Health, 3,* 67-111.

Chapter 8

# Family Health Practice with Older Adult Populations

Christine A. Price
Francis K. O. Yuen

## *INTRODUCTION*

Industrialized nations are, for the first time in the history, experiencing a dramatic increase in the life expectancy of both men and women. In the United States, at the beginning of the twentieth century, life expectancy was estimated at forty-six years for men and forty-nine years for women (Zarit and Eggebeen, 1995). In contrast, at the turn of the twenty-first century, life expectancy had risen to seventy-two years for men and seventy-nine for women. This increased longevity is one of a number of demographic factors that have contributed to the rapid growth of the aging population (Atchley, 2000; Kinsella, 1996).

Additional factors that have contributed to the expanding population of elders include improved medical technology (the use of antibiotics, effective treatment of disease, preventative measures), steady decline in birth rates, and improved sanitation and food preservation methods. When the first U.S. Census was conducted in 1790, only 2 percent (50,000) of the 2.5 million Americans living at that time were sixty-five years of age or older. One hundred years later, that number had risen to 2.4 million older adults, constituting 4 percent of the U.S. population. By the year 2000, the population of adults sixty-five years of age and older measured 34.7 million, constituting 12.6 percent of the U.S. population (Atchley, 2000). These numbers are predicted to increase further to 39.7 million by 2010 and 70.3 million by 2030 (Administration on Aging, 2002).

Many implications of these demographic changes for the aging family arise, for example, multigenerational interaction and the opportunity to provide care to aging family members. In addition, new family structures are being created, such as the "beanpole" family, which consists of multiple generations living at one time with fewer family members in each generation (Bengtson, Rosenthal, and Burton, 1995; Dwyer, Folts, and Rosenberg, 1994). This change in family structure is a direct result of both increased life expectancy and declining fertility rates.

Within the family and larger society, increased longevity has brought about expanded interest and concern over the social issue of providing care to aging family members. Researchers examining the sources of assistance provided to older adults report that 80 percent of care provided to aging family members comes from their immediate family network (Coward, Horne, and Dwyer, 1992; Dwyer, Folts, and Rosenberg, 1994). The term *family caregiving* is often used to describe the instrumental, emotional, and sometimes financial assistance provided by family members for older individuals. The motivational factors behind caregiving behaviors include (1) love and affection, (2) reciprocation for past assistance, and (3) feelings of filial responsibility (Dwyer, 1996).

Aging family members may be cared for within the family; however, usually one individual, labeled the *primary caregiver,* provides regular, hands-on assistance with daily activities, coordinates supplemental care, and serves as an intermediary between the older adult and social service and benefits agencies (Atchley, 2000; Dwyer, 1996; Zarit and Eggebeen, 1995). The likelihood of becoming a primary caregiver largely depends on other available family members, geographic closeness to the older adult, the extent of employment of caregiver candidates, and most important, gender. Caregiving responsibilities are largely the domain of women because the nurturing nature of caregiving is thought to be the work of women, because women's employment is often viewed as expendable, and because women are socialized to be altruistic and emotionally invested in their familial roles (Dwyer, 1996). As a result, women provide a disproportionate amount of care to aging family members in both spousal and adult-child capacities.

In addition to the social context of the family, researchers have identified a caregiving hierarchy that families inadvertently follow when an older family member requires care. First, if a spouse is available, he or she is likely to become the primary source of care. If a spouse is not present or is unable to provide care, an adult child, most often an adult daughter, is the next person expected to assume responsibility. Finally, when an adult child is unavailable to provide care, another female relative is the most likely candidate for primary caregiver (Dwyer, 1996; Zarit and Eggebeen, 1995).

A considerable number of researchers have documented the burden associated with caregiving responsibilities, most specifically the impact of this stress on the emotional and physical health of caregivers. Findings indicate that being a caregiver is strongly associated with increased susceptibility to depression, lower measures of well-being, increased emotional distress, and increased likelihood for health problems (Zarit and Eggebeen, 1995). Reports of stress do increase in certainly family caregiving situations, for example, having an aging parent with emotional or behavioral problems that require consistent care. In addition, the diagnosis of dementia or other cognitive incapacities also enhances the challenges experienced by caregivers.

In addition to stressors related to the physical or mental status of the elder, conflict with other family members is another source of stress that caregivers often report. Commonly, caregivers report conflict with family about the illness of the aging parent, decisions concerning treatment, and the extent of support and involvement of other family members (Zarit and Eggebeen, 1995). At the same time, situations outside of the family, such as work-related problems and reduced opportunities for recreational pursuits or personal time, also contribute to caregiver burden.

To provide support to caregivers of aging family members, it is important to recognize the family context in which caregiving responsibilities are taking place. Each family has a cultural environment, created as a result of communication and interaction patterns, which will significantly influence any response to a caregiving crisis. The resources available to family members and the types of assistance exchanged between family members will also vary widely and be influenced by factors external to the family. Just as with any other type of family intervention, it is imperative that those providing support recognize and attempt to work within the existing family environment, as well as the current resources available.

This chapter discusses some of the intervention considerations and skills in working with older adults and their families.

## CASE STUDY: THE MARTINEZ FAMILY

### Father

Manuel is a Hispanic American who, in his seventies, is showing signs of early dementia. Manuel is very forgetful; he becomes easily disoriented and recently got lost on his way home from the local supermarket. Although his wife, Maria, is not a manipulative woman, she has been able to hide many of her husband's dementia symptoms. As a result, it is only when Manuel is taken out of the familiarity of his home that his confusion becomes much more obvious. Recently, Manuel's daughter, Carmen, began to realize the extent of her father's advancing dementia when she stopped by after work and her father insisted that the neighbors, who had lived next door for twenty-three years, had just moved in yesterday. The Martinez family has been living in the same house in Cleveland, Ohio, for more than three decades. To further complicate matters, Manuel has a short temper and becomes angry and verbally abusive when anyone suggests he is confused or may need some assistance. He is strongly against any "strangers" entering his home and providing care to him or his wife. He views family support to be the responsibility of his daughters, specifically Carmen.

### Mother

Maria came to the United States as a teenager from rural Mexico and now is in her late sixties. She has raised five children, two having died (one as a child and one in his teen years as a result of a drive-by shooting). Maria is a passive woman who still mourns her dead children and periodically has severe depressive episodes. She does not have any friends of her own and depends entirely on her daughter Carmen for all of her emotional needs. Maria has chronic arthritis, which severely limits her mobility and capacity to care for herself and her husband. She has always left the decisions and responsibilities to her husband Manuel, who is viewed as the patriarch of the family. Maria has never questioned or confronted Manuel about anything, primarily because she feels it is not her place and because she is fearful of his quick temper. She has been aware of Manuel's confusion and growing forgetfulness for the past two years but has done her best to hide these symptoms from her children. She is afraid of what may happen should the children discover his declining faculties. Ultimately, Maria is frightened that Manuel will require more care than she can provide and as a result will need to be placed in a nursing home. This thought is something she is unable to deal with, so as a result, she denies and purposefully hides his growing confusion. In addition, Maria is also in complete denial about her own physical limitations and the reality that she may eventually need more assistance herself.

### *Adult Children*

The three remaining children in the Martinez family are Anita, Roberto, and Carmen. One daughter, Anita, lives in New York and rarely comes home but does keep in touch with the family through regular phone calls. The middle child and only son, Roberto, also lives out of state in Indiana. He views himself as the next generation's patriarch of the family. However, it is his wife who maintains contact with the family and then keeps him informed. The only time Roberto becomes involved is when significant decisions regarding the family need to be made. He makes these types of decisions without any discussion with his sisters.

The oldest daughter, Carmen, is the primary caregiver in this family. She lives near her parents and stops by regularly to check on them. In addition to being a caregiver, Carmen is married with two small children (ages four and six) and has a part-time job to supplement her husband's income. Often Carmen feels overwhelmed with her sense of responsibility to her parents as well as to her family of procreation. To add additional pressure, her husband (Juan) gets angry with her when she spends a great deal of time at her parents' house. He resents her caregiving role and is constantly voicing his displeasure with her siblings' lack of involvement.

Carmen is becoming increasingly aware of her father's growing limitations; however, her mother consistently denies any problems and dismisses Carmen's concerns. Carmen's brother, Roberto, says his father sounds fine when he speaks with him on the phone and criticizes her for overreacting. Anita is too far away to be of much help and says only that she will support whatever Carmen decides to do, thereby leaving the responsibilities to Carmen.

## *ASSESSMENT AND DIAGNOSTIC IMPRESSIONS*

1. Manuel has early stage dementia and will need increased supervision and assistance.
2. Maria is in denial about her husband's decline and has very low self-perception and little experience living independently. Her health limitations and depression need to be assessed and treated. It is likely she will need assistance in providing care to her husband.
3. Both Manuel and Maria are reluctant clients who need support and incentive to become more receptive to receiving services.
4. Carmen has competing responsibilities between her own family and her parents' needs. She feels frustrated about the limited support she is receiving from her siblings and resentful that these responsibilities must fall on her shoulders.
5. Roberto and Anita need to become more involved and aware of their parents' situation.
6. A dramatic lack of communication exists in this family. All family members enable Maria's weakness and Manuel's need for control. Carmen's personal and family boundaries need to be recognized.
7. The extended Martinez family is participating in the renegotiation of the relationships among its family members. The social worker and other service providers are to facilitate this negotiation process.
8. Family interactions in the Martinez family are the primary sources of meaning as well as the bases and consequences of their behaviors. They are, therefore, the sources of power to produce and sustain changes. For this reason, family interactions are the most important aspect and the focus of any human service interventions to the Martinez family.

## PROBLEM SOURCES AND MANIFESTATIONS

The health conditions of Manuel, the restricted sense of self and the history of depression of Maria, the disconnections of two adult children, and the overwhelmedness of Carmen are the major presenting problems. The changing nature and function of the Martinez family due to the changes in health and the interrelatedness of family members are some of the critical underlying issues for this family.

The hierarchical and gender-specific role expectations and family rules have affected the communication and enabled codependence among family members. This family is facing major transitions and challenges which have threatened the basic family rules and practice that have been in working order for this family and have not required any adjustment until now.

In many ways, Manuel and Maria have been a functional system that has maintained a great degree of balance. Since Manuel's health decline, Carmen has become the major source of input and support to the system and keeps it from collapsing. For Carmen, to function as the family caregiver is an energy-draining and time-consuming role that requires too much output and commitment from her with very little replenishment or relief.

## INTERVENTION SKILLS

1. A mental status examination and diagnosis are needed for Manuel to determine his mental functioning, particularly the extent of his dementia.

2. Manuel also needs to receive a medical diagnosis and a treatment plan to provide the family with medically realistic expectations and to develop a plan of care for the family.

3. Contact local area agencies on aging to ascertain what support programs are available in the community to assist Carmen with providing care to her parents, for example, home-delivered meals, available home health services, respite care services, adult day care programs, and so forth.

4. Meet individually with Maria to assist her with areas of self-confidence, encouragement in taking care of herself, and dealing with her depressive episodes.

5. Arrange for Maria to attend a caregiver support group so that she can meet other caregivers (preferably spousal) and also make personal social contacts of her own.

6. Meet individually with Carmen to address her pattern of enabling her parents' dependence and her father's control. She can learn ways to establish and maintain her own boundaries while demanding assistance from her siblings. Enrollment in training or workshops such as self-care or assertiveness could be arranged. Carmen could also attend a caregiver support group to identify with other caregivers in her same position.

7. Arrange a family meeting that includes a medical doctor as well as a social worker to make plans for the future care of Manuel as he continues to decline. It is important that this family does not wait until another crisis point before decisions are made. Decisions need to be made regarding the potential placement of Manuel or the arrangement of in-home services for Manuel and Maria for as long as possible. Facilities that have dementia units specializing in the care of seniors with dementia need to be located and toured by family members. Manuel's name may need to be placed on a waiting list, depending on his prognosis and the popularity of the facility. Should Manuel need to be placed in a care facility, decisions concerning the care of Maria also need to be made, obviously with her input as to whether she wants (and reasonably can) remain in the family home alone or if she would prefer to relocate to a retirement community with other seniors.

8. The social worker should be cognizant of the Hispanic cultural backgrounds of the Martinez family. The different degrees of acculturation to the urban American culture and the various extents of adherence to specific Hispanic cultural practices by the Martinez family and each of its members are all important clinical variables. Culturally competent practice that respects and is in tune with the Martinez family is the first step toward any possible clinical alliance and success. It is most likely that the use of metaphor will be an effective approach for the Martinez family. Metaphors, particularly those that have cultural relevance, help clients grasp meanings, understand problems, and envision alternative outcomes. They can also be used to plant seed ideas or suggest changes.

9. Voluntarily or involuntarily, members of the Martinez family are likely candidates for becoming the reluctant clients. A family health

social worker should respect the family's rights to self-determination while attempting to identify ways to promote the family's self-efficacy and proper understanding of the family's situations and choices. Rooney (1992) discusses various strategies in working with involuntary clients. The social worker can help members of the Martinez family reframe the situation and attribute alternative reasons to reduce dissonance. Foot-in-the-door methods should also be considered to generate incremental changes and to facilitate self-attribution for changes. The intention is not to change clients' behaviors immediately; instead, the attention should be on helping them clarify their firmly held central values and explore new insights. Role revision is an effective approach that can bring about new insight and perspectives.

10. The family health social worker should also try to assist Manuel and Maria to evaluate their current situation. This includes helping them see the unanticipated or self-defeating consequences of inaction or action and consider alternatives in meeting their goals while remaining mindful of the constraints. For example, "I see the inconsistency and I am concerned because you are trying to achieve (the desired result), but your (behaviors, actions, attitudes, or inaction) contradict that and are likely to create (possible negative consequence)."

11. Conduct family counseling to improve communication within the family and to provide family members with strategies on how to work with and potentially confront Manuel, especially concerning the increased need for support services and possible placement. Family meetings need to take place as frequently as once a week, with the out-of-state siblings participating at least via the telephone.

12. A family health social worker may assess the clinical appropriateness and consider a variety of family practice approaches for the Martinez family. The application of these therapeutic approaches, however, should first consider Manuel's health and mental health conditions as well as the readiness and willingness of all family members. Following is a review of such family practice approaches.

    a. Structural family therapy (Minuchin, 1974; Haley, 1976; Aponte, 1976) aims to reorganize the family into a more functional structure by challenging the family's view of the problem and expanding its options for response. This therapy approach also tries to alter the family's interactions to clarify boundaries and authority.

b. To address the issue of inadequate differentiation among family members, a social worker may borrow skills from Murray Bowen's (1961) intergenerational family therapy, which focuses on the degrees of emotional "stuck-togetherness" of family members. The aim is to assist the Martinez family members to recognize the patterns and to understand the family legacy. Particularly for Maria and Carmen, the social worker has to assist them to be aware of their feelings of guilt and that they are free to change their own behaviors.

c. Virginia Satir's (1972) communication and experiential approach may call for the use of a family sculpting that facilitates family members to gain new understanding and experience. An example is to ask the Martinez family members to physically rearrange themselves to illustrate how they relate to one another.

d. The adoption of the cognitive-behavioral therapeutic approach may apply cognitive restructuring to assist Maria, Manuel, and Carmen in their understanding of their situations. Applying the social learning theory, the social worker should consider additional learning opportunities for the family members to gain new coping skills to address their unique needs.

e. To address the issue of the changing family and its members, the social worker may adopt the social constructionist approach to assist the Martinez family in their search for new meanings for their situations. Using the narrative approach, the social worker listens to client-generated stories and helps the clients (Manuel, Maria, and Carmen) restructure the stories and explore new possibilities. By engaging the Martinezes to author the next chapter of their family legacy, the social worker empowers the family and each individual member to set goals and make plans for the future.

Although many approaches for family therapy exist, many of them share common theoretical bases and skills. Most of the approaches for family therapy focus on changing people's here-and-now interactions with others. The concern is not with what caused a problem but with what seems to maintain it.

## EVALUATION

From the write-up of the psychosocial assessment to the uses of genogram and ecomap, a family health social worker applies appropriate family and individual assessment tools to set the baselines for the design of interventions. The overall needs of the Martinez family and the unique needs of each individual member are to be clearly identified and defined. The development of treatment plans sets the goals and objectives for the interventions as well as for the focus of evaluations.

The family health social worker will measure both the process and the outcome of the interventions. Data collection can be achieved through formal assessments by established scales, observations, interviews, and other methods. After a certain period of time of service or after the settlement of any critical changes of the Martinez family situation, the social worker will assess the impact of the services on the family and its members.

Single-subject designs can be applied to assess the progress of Manuel, Marie, or Carmen toward their individual goals and provide valuable data for service improvement. Qualitative data from observations, progress notes, or comments from the Martinez family could be included in the evaluation of the effectiveness and efficiency of the services and their delivery.

## REFERENCES

Administration on Aging (2002). *A profile of older Americans: 2001, Future growth*. Available online: <http://www.aoa.dhhs.gov/aoa/STATS/profile/2001/2.html.

Aponte, H. (1976). Underorganization and the poor family. In P. Guerin. (Ed.), *Family therapy: Theory and practice*. New York: Gardner Press.

Atchley, R. C. (2000). *Social forces of aging*. Belmont, CA: Wadsworth.

Bengtson, V., Rosenthal, C., and Burton, L. (1995). Paradoxes of families and aging. In R. H. Bainstock and L. K. George (Eds.), *Handbook of aging and the social sciences* (pp. 253-282). San Diego, CA: Academic Press.

Bowen, M. (1961). Family pschotherapy. *American Journal of Orthopsychiatry, 31*, 40-60.

Coward, R. T., Horne, C., and Dwyer, J. W. (1992). Demographic perspectives on gender and family caregiving. In J. S. Dwyer and R. T. Coward (Eds.), *Gender families and elder care* (pp. 18-33). Newbury Park, CA: Sage.

Dwyer, J. W. (1996). The effects of illness on the family. In R. Blieszner and V. H. Bedford (Eds.), *Aging and the family* (pp. 401-421). Westport, CT: Praeger.

Dwyer, J. W., Folts, W. E., and Rosenberg, E. (1994). Caregiving in a social context. *Educational Gerontology, 20,* 615-631.

Haley, J. (1976). *Problem solving therapy: New strategies for effective family therapy.* San Francisco: Jossey-Bass.

Kinsella, K. (1996). Aging and the family: Present and future. In J. S. Dwyer and R. T. Coward (Eds.), *Gender families and elder care* (pp. 32-56). Newbury Park, CA: Sage.

Minuchin, S. (1974). *Families and family therapy.* Cambridge, MA: Harvard University Press.

Rooney, R. (1992). *Strategies for work with involuntary clients.* New York: Columbia University Press.

Satir, V. (1972). *Peoplemaking.* Palo Alto: Science and Behavior Books.

Zarit, S. H. and Eggebeen, D. J. (1995). Parent-child relationships in adulthood and old age. In M. H. Bornstein (Ed.), *Handbook of parenting,* Volume 1 (pp. 119-140). Mahwah, NJ: Lawrence Erlbaum.

Chapter 9

# Navigating Family Health in Families with Alcohol Abuse

James G. Daley

This chapter describes the current models of family recovery from alcohol abuse and how the family health social work practice (FHSWP) model is adapted to family recovery issues. The chapter concludes with a discussion of future directions for FHSWP with families with alcohol abuse.

## *INTRODUCTION*

Alcohol abuse is devastating to a family system, producing a substance-centered pattern that thwarts appropriate individual growth and maturity, produces pathological family behaviors, and involves a fluctuating abuse pattern that leave family members shell-shocked and resistant to hope (Collins, Leonard, and Searles, 1990; Freeman, 1993; Brown and Lewis, 1995; Curtis, 1999). The role of the family in the treatment process has ranged from being peripheral to being a major causal and destructive force to needing concurrent or separate treatment irrespective of the recovery path of the alcohol abuser (Rivers, 1994; Nowinski, 1999). Treatment and recovery emphasis has evolved from a "singular focus on the alcoholic," to evolving support systems such as Al-Anon, to working on "codependence" and "adult children of alcoholics," to growing understanding of the complexities in families navigating substance abuse (Brown and Lewis, 1995, p. 280). The pathways of recovery for families are more complex and not directly correlated to the individual substance abuser's recovery. In sum, family recovery is a clinical and research issue worthy of exploration.

## MODELS OF FAMILY RECOVERY FROM ALCOHOL ABUSE

Several models have been suggested for capturing a family's recovery process from alcoholism. Unfortunately, as can be seen in Table 9.1, the research to date has focused on alcoholism rather than explanatory models that differentiate alcoholism from other substance abuse or highlight distinct difference between family recovery from alcoholism as compared to cocaine dependence or methamphetamine

TABLE 9.1. Models of Family Recovery from Alcoholism

| Model | Reference | Stages |
| --- | --- | --- |
| Adaptation model | Jackson, 1954; Rivers, 1994 | Avoid or deny problem; social isolation and family centered on alcoholism; family disorganization and helplessness; spouse takes control and family stabilizes without alcoholic's role; family leaves alcoholic; family established without alcoholic; recovery and reunion with alcoholic |
| Process model | Rosenberg, 1981-1982 | Random phase; recrimination phase; policing phase; realization phase |
| Developmental model | Gorski and Miller, 1986; Curtis, 1999 | Pretreatment stage; stabilization stage; early recovery stage; middle recovery stage; late recovery stage; maintenance/remission stage |
| Phase model | Steinglass, 1987 | Early phase (accommodate or challenge); middle phase (homeostasis centered on alcoholism); late phase (pathways: stable wet dependent, stable wet or controlled use nondependent, stable dry dependent, stable dry nondependent) |
| Emotional systems model | Treadway, 1989 | Disengagement; differentiation; negotiation; conflict management; intimacy |
| "Taking charge" model | Schlesinger and Horberg, 1994 | Getting started; strengthening the family; confronting the addiction; thriving as a family |
| Recovery model | Brown and Lewis, 1995; Brown and Lewis, 1999 | Drinking stage; transition stage ("trauma of recovery"); early recovery stage; ongoing recovery stage |

dependence. Further research is needed to explore the similarities and differences between families navigating different substance abuse. Is the process generalizable for all drugs or are there distinctly different paths for different drug recovery? We have no answer to that question. Concurrently, primary research was undertaken with male alcoholics with little differentiation between family recovery processes for female alcoholics as contrasted to male alcoholics. Likewise, no research has occurred differentiating same-sex partners and families, or any extensive research on differentiating family recovery for substance abuse by ethnicity or culture. In sum, the research reported is promising but bounded in utility by these flaws.

Within these flaws, seven models have been proposed for family recovery.

### Jackson's Seven-Stage Adaptation Model

One of the first family recovery models was developed from a three-year study of Al-Anon wives by Jackson (1954). From this study, Jackson proposed a seven-stage process. The first stage, *avoid or deny problem,* occurs when the family initially minimizes the escalating problem. "It's not that bad" or "It will get better when his job is less stressful" are common comments made during this phase. The second stage, *social isolation and family centered on alcoholism,* occurs when the family recognizes that the alcohol abuse is rampant, withdraws from social contact, and ineffectively tries to eliminate the alcohol abuse by harassment or hiding alcohol. "This has got to stop!" or "We'll work this out. We just need to help him more" are common comments made during this phase. The third stage, *family disorganization and helplessness,* is a chaotic time during which the family becomes angry or desperate as they realize their efforts will not fix the issue. The alcoholic family member is rejected, children in the family often exhibit behavioral outbursts, marital tension soars, and the alcoholism is less likely to be kept as a social secret. "I've had it!" or "He's tearing this family apart" are common comments during this phase. The fourth stage, *spouse takes control and family stabilizes without alcoholic's role,* occurs when the nonalcoholic spouse accepts the central role of stabilizer and begins to exclude the alcoholic from family responsibilities. This stage can produce intense reactivity from the alcoholic who wants to maintain the illusion of normal parental position while still centered on alcohol intake and discovers an increasingly exclusionary family. Family members often seek support groups such as Al-Anon during this stage. "I've realized that he's not going to change" or "It's his choice whether to come back or not" are typical comments in this stage. The fifth stage, *family leaves alcoholic,* occurs when the family emotionally and sometimes physically leaves the alcoholic. In a natural progression from the fourth stage, the family settles into a routine without the alcoholic and has no expectations for the alcoholic's involvement. "He's no longer part of this family" or "We've got to get on with our lives" are common comments in this stage. The sixth stage, *family established without alcoholic,* continues that separation from the alcoholic and solidifies the family as exclusive of the alcoholic. Family rules and processes become established that eliminate the alcoholic from the family. "He's not welcome here" or "He's got his life; we've got ours" are common comments in this stage. Many families, according to Jackson, do not progress past this stage as the final stage requires recovery efforts on the part of the substance abuser. The seventh stage, *recovery and reunion with alcoholic,* occurs when the alcoholic discontinues alcohol abuse, begins personal recovery efforts, and seeks reunification with the family. This stage is very tense, filled with mistrust by the family and remorse by the alcoholic, and is difficult to navigate successfully. Families have stabilized without the alcoholic and may resist trying again with the alcoholic. "It's too late" or "He'll just go back to drinking" are common comments in this stage.

Jackson's stages are useful to conceptualize the family's journey but have had no empirical research done to verify that the stages exist, that families progress in this sequence, or whether multiple paths to recovery occur in addition to or alongside this sequence. The distinction of the Jackson model was that it occurred in the 1950s when much attention was centered on individual recovery strategies and few researchers were looking at the family's process. As Seilhamer (1991) asserts, "although written over 35 years ago, Jackson's representation of alcoholic families continues to be cited as relevant for today's families that have a substance-abusing member" (p. 175).

### Rosenberg's Four-Phase Process Model

The Rosenberg model (1981-1982) describes the family recovery process as four phases of therapy. The first phase, the *random phase,* is the initial process in therapy when families are uncertain why they are in therapy, minimize or deny the problem at times, or avoid looking at any family role in the issue. The random phase can feel chaotic or unproductive in that families are resistant to work on the issues. The second phase, the *recrimination phase,* involves family members describing the worst events during the alcoholism in an effort to get the therapist to side with the family against the alcoholic. The third phase, the *policing phase,* is a phase in which families challenge the boundaries of treatment by missing appointments or undermining agreed-upon treatment goals. This challenging time is an attempt to focus attention on the treatment parameters so as to avoid beginning the work of recovery. The final phase, the *realization phase,* occurs when the family ceases testing the therapist or avoiding the issues and begins to work on the impact of alcoholism on the family. The therapist is finally able to work with family members through their anger and hurt, and encourage development of a healthier and more adaptive family system.

The Rosenberg model is a useful reminder of the rapid reactivity of alcoholism-damaged families in the early stages of treatment. No empirical studies exist to verify that the phases actually occur in that order or consist of those issues. Therefore, the primary utility of this model is as a conceptual tool for steeling oneself as a therapist for the bumpy road of treatment of the family with alcohol abuse.

### Curtis's Six-Stage Developmental Model

The next model was adapted by Curtis (1999) from Gorski and Miller's (1986) model for individual recovery. Curtis proposed six developmental stages of recovery for the family. The first stage, the *pretreatment stage,* occurs with a crisis, whether from an overwhelming event (sexual misconduct, an alcoholic blackout alarming enough to demand action, etc.) or a climaxing of chronic tension and uncertainty. In whatever manner the situation unfolds, the family has reached a moment of determination to get help. This "motivational crisis" (Curtis, 1999, p. 117) initiates the treatment process. The second stage, the *stabilization stage,* is when basic education on substance abuse and the family is provided, clarification is emphasized between the family's responsibility (e.g., enabling) and that for which the family is not responsible (the addiction). A combination of treatment and support group involvement usually is set up in this stage.

The third stage, the *early recovery stage,* is a tough time; in this stage the issues of family structure during the addiction and the beginnings of a recovery family structure are negotiated and clarified. A painful relearning process occurs in which new roles unfold and old, dysfunctional behaviors are challenged. The fourth stage, the *middle recovery stage,* is when the family "begins to rebuild self-image and self-esteem and to establish a personal structured recovery plan" (p. 118). The family begins to emerge as a new entity with more effective coping skills for navigating relapse or continued use by the alcoholic. If the alcoholic is not in recovery, this stage can be very difficult for the alcoholic and sometimes might prompt the alcoholic to seek treatment or act out. The fifth stage, the *late recovery stage,* centers on family members working through longer-term issues such as family-of-origin or intimacy concerns. The focus moves from how to handle the alcohol-abusing behavior to lifestyles and goals. The final stage, the *maintenance/remission stage,* focuses on "lifelong recovery through continued personal growth" (p. 118). Issues of personal potential and maturation are the primary focus.

The Curtis model focuses on an ideal progression toward the ideal maturation, far beyond most managed care funding frameworks but potentially achievable within some support groups that people attend for a lifetime. As with Maslow's hierarchy, the Curtis model has value as an ideal end point for which to aim. No empirical research has been done to verify that families progress in the sequence, what proportion of families ever go beyond the third stage, or whether personal maturation has any impact on the alcoholic's recovery. In other words, if family members mature and are healthy while the alcoholic spirals toward early death, is this recovery model useful? Can family recovery be disconnected from the substance abuser, or is "full recovery" achievable only if recovery includes a successfully recovering alcoholic?

### *Steinglass's Three-Phase Model*

Steinglass (1987) describes a model that explains how substance abuse impacts the developmental phases of the family and how a family can travel one of four pathways. The first phase, the *early phase,* focuses on how the family initially reacts to the alcoholic behavior and indicates that families typically either accommodate or challenge the behavior. If a family is newly forming then the family identity, boundaries, and communication style can be distorted. Family rules and intimacy issues can be damaged and the family system becomes centered on the alcoholism. Conversely, the newly forming family intolerant of the alcoholic behavior would challenge the behavior and potentially dissolve the family unit. The second phase, the *middle phase,* occurs when the family creates homeostasis centered around alcoholism. A stability occurs as the family seeks to minimize the impact of the alcoholism on the family by developing rigid rules and accommodating the alcoholic behavior. Stability overrules any long-term developmental needs and families often get stuck in an unhealthy ritual of denial, accommodation, and sacrifice of family member needs. The last phase, the *late phase,* consists of established family pathways that can be healthy or rigidly destructive. Steinglass describes four pathways. The "stable wet dependent family" accommodates to the alcoholism and has developed family structure centered on enabling continued substance abuse. The "stable wet or controlled use nondependent family" is the family that is beginning to confront and reclaim family structure from the substance abuse, yet the alcoholic might be still using or has reduced using alcohol. The "stable dry dependent family" is the family in which the alcoholic is no longer using but the system is still centered on the potential for relapse and the issues surrounding alcoholism as the primary family structure. This type of family could be considered the "dry drunk family"; nothing has changed except alcohol intake. The final path is the "stable dry nondependent family" in which the alcohol use has stopped, the recovery process is occurring, and the individuals are involved in major family restructuring.

Steinglass's model is useful to highlight how alcohol abuse can damage normal family development and how families can stay stuck in dysfunctional family structures. No empirical research has verified that these model phases actually occur as described, and the pathways are limited in utility as they do not provide as detailed a description of the family's process of recovery as other models described in this chapter.

### *Treadway's Five-Stage Emotional Systems Model*

Treadway (1989) has a five-stage model that focuses on family recovery. The first stage, *disengagement,* seeks to "shift the responsibility for the drinking behavior back to the drinker and to help the spouse discontinue her standard responses to the substance abuse" (p. 38). This stage involves a paradigm shift from being stuck in the alcoholism-focused system to setting limits on the control of alcohol on the family system. The second stage, *differentiation,* seeks to "help the family tolerate discomfort and confusion with sobriety and to reduce expectations about early recovery" (p. 80). Assuming rapid family health in early recovery produces unrealistic and easily dashed expectations. As the recovery work begins, the family is encouraged to expect and cope with the discomfort of fluctuating change efforts. The third stage, *negotiation,* seeks to "teach the marital partners negotiating and problem-solving skills that will enhance their sense of competence and their ability to work together" (p. 84). As the family progresses in recovery, the partners have to shift their problem-solving efforts from avoidance or blackmail to negotiation and direct communication. This stage serves as an educational arena for change. The fourth stage, *conflict management,* occurs when the partners are learning how to "tolerate conflict," "fight fairly," and "tolerate unresolved conflict without allowing it to escalate out of control" (p. 88). Education and resolution of family issues combine to facilitate family functioning. The final stage, *intimacy,* targets "a balance of closeness and distance" as the final recovery arena (p. 95). As differentiation, negotiation, and conflict management skills are developed, the delicate issue of enhancing intimacy can occur.

Treadway's model is based on clinical experience and has not had empirical research conducted to confirm the model's validity. It is unproven empirically whether the suggested sequence of stages is the most effective framework, if the issues suggested in the model are accurate, or if a direct link exists between these stages and effective alcoholism family recovery. The model's emphasis on developing basic skills before working on family intimacy seems noteworthy as a sequence.

## *Schlesinger and Horberg's Four-Stage "Taking Charge" Model*

Schlesinger and Horberg (1994) have developed what they call a four-stage "taking charge" model of family recovery. The first stage, *getting started,* focuses on getting the family to disengage from the addiction and to decide to change their family structure. However, before confronting the addiction, Schlesinger and Horberg advocate that the family must go through a *strengthening the family* stage where the family shifts from feeling emotionally drained and desperate to feeling recharged and ready to work on the issues. If family members confronted the addiction in the first stage, they would likely feel overwhelmed and handle the task inadequately. Therefore the transition strengthening stage is needed to prepare the family. The third stage involves *confronting the addiction:* the family directly discusses the addiction, perhaps through an intervention, and commits to discontinuing unhealthy behaviors that enable the addictive behavior to be in charge of the family. The family begins to "take charge" of the position the addiction serves in the family. The final stage facilitates *thriving as a family.* Letting go of the trauma of the addiction and the need for retribution releases energy that can be used in healthy family functioning. Although being realistic about the ebb and flow of recovery and the different variations of recovery, the family aims toward family enhancing goals.

The Schlesinger and Horberg model aptly encourages building family strength before dealing with the addiction. No empirical research exists to verify this model or to support the proposed sequencing.

### Brown and Lewis's Four-Stage Recovery Model

The final model to discuss is the family recovery model proposed by Brown and Lewis (1995). The model was developed from the Family Recovery Project at the Mental Research Institute in Palo Alto, California. The Family Recovery Project sought to study the "normal processes of recovery, over time, for the family in which one or both have stopped drinking" (p. 279). From the family interviews, they developed a four-stage family recovery model. The first stage, the *drinking stage,* occurs when alcohol is "the central organizing principle of the family system, controlling and dictating family beliefs, behaviors, and development" and the family faces the double bind of rationalizing the substance abuse while denying its devastation (p. 284). Treatment during the drinking stage focuses on challenging the alcoholic family system, encouraging individual emotional separation from the alcohol-centered system, and offering support in recognizing the effect of alcohol on family system. The second stage, the *transition stage,* usually is prompted by a crisis in or overwhelming demand on the family. An arrest, a blackout, a violent act, or some event tears away the denial and reveals the need for recovery. This stage is marked by abstinence and "the trauma of recovery" (p. 288). Unable to continue the denial but uncertain how to navigate the new family structure, families struggle with how to function. The substance abuser and the family members are often at different stages of individual recovery and "the collapse of the system is necessary for family recovery" (p. 289). Treatment in the transition stage includes challenging the core beliefs of the old system, acknowledging that family life is out of control, and emphasizing the importance of individual recovery. Families can dissolve during this stage—a stage that is considered extremely painful for individuals and family. The third stage, the *early recovery stage,* "is characterized by steady abstinence and the integration of new thinking, attitudes, and behaviors" (p. 296) and emphasizes "the need for emotional separation, the need for a focus on the individuals, and the importance of not rushing too quickly to patch up a family system" (p. 301). Support groups and education are vital to help families navigate this stage. Treatment in the early recovery stage includes encouraging behavior and cognitive change, watching for signs of relapse, and working on trauma resolution. Family functioning is discussed, but the primary focus continues to be on individual recovery issues. The final stage, the *ongoing recovery stage,* focuses on "finding a balance between individual and couple and family growth" (p. 306). Because the family is "less crisis organized and crisis dominated and there is less, if any, regular trauma and instability," the focus of treatment emphasizes "healthy family growth based on solid individual recovery" (pp. 306, 309).

The Brown and Lewis family recovery model offers a sequential process of recovery. In fact, their treatment approach asserts that "we can now offer them a map of what lies ahead and, particularly, what is normal and expected over a long-term process of change and new development" (Brown and Lewis, 1995, p. 301). Their research involved extensive interviews with families in ongoing recovery and focused on anecdotal descriptions of what stages they went through. The stages are based on these data but have not had extensive empirical research to validate the hypothesized process.

## Common Elements from the Models of Family Recovery

The seven models describe linear processes progressing from active substance use and an alcoholism-centered family process to a healthier family via various forms of confrontation, education, and traumatic separation from pathological family structures. All models highlight the importance of individual recovery and support groups. Few of the models had any empirical research upon which to base their models. Similarities exist conceptually between the models, yet many elements of family health are not emphasized or are underrepresented in the discussion of family recovery. One model that might enhance the discussion of family recovery is family health social work practice.

## FAMILY HEALTH SOCIAL WORK PRACTICE AND FAMILY RECOVERY ISSUES

An emphasis on family health has been explored in many arenas. Areas of social work intervention include family-centered practice (Cole, 1995; Hartman and Laird, 1983; Kelley, 1996; Laird, 1995; Powell, 1996), family-based services (Pecora et al., 1995), family preservation (Denby, Curtis, and Alford, 1998; Faria, 1994; Ronnau and Marlow, 1993; Wells and Beigel, 1991), family practice (Pinderhughes, 1995; Vosler, 1996), family support services (Comer and Fraser, 1998; Lightburn and Kemp, 1994), family strengths approach (Duncan and Brown, 1992; Weick and Saleebey, 1995; Werrbach, 1996), community-centered family services (Sviridoff and Ryan, 1997), family problem solving (Reid, 1985), social work with families (Munson, 1980), and family health social work practice (Pardeck and Yuen, 1997; Pardeck et al., 1998; Weick, 1986; Weick and Saleebey, 1995). Each of these approaches highlights to varying degrees the importance and complexity of maintaining family health during difficult personal or family crises (e.g. child abuse, life threatening illness, natural disaster).

One approach with particular potential is family health social work practice. This approach builds on previous research and theory on family health, and asserts that seven dimensions combine to facilitate family health (Pardeck and Yuen, 1999). Family health is defined as a state of holistic well-being of the family system. Family health is manifested by the development of, and continuous interaction among, the physical, mental, emotional, social, economic, cultural and spiritual dimensions of the family, which results in the holistic well-being of the family and its members. (Pardeck and Yuen, 1999, p. 1)

These seven dimensions, similar to seven "pistons" on a "family engine," must work in cooperation. When one or more begin to fail, the engine runs badly and finally fails completely.

The models of substance-abusing family recovery acknowledge that family functioning is distorted and destructive to family members when the family is alcohol centered. The family health model asserts that the seven dimensions are distorted as the economic health, the spiritual health, the physical health, and so forth are weakened by the abusive cycle of alcoholism. The holistic well-being of the family members is impaired.

The models of family recovery from alcohol abuse describe recovery as beginning with abstinence and confrontation of the damaging and destructive pattern of enabling that is common in families with active alcohol abuse. Individual recovery predates family recovery. Family recovery is undergirded by support groups and extra-familial assistance. Families are considered healthy when couple and family growth emerges within an environment of trust and intimacy. Alcoholism is restrained through abstinence and vigilance while families cautiously reconnect with each other.

The models of family recovery from alcohol abuse illustrate the recovery efforts related to alcohol abuse containment and reestablishment of family function. However, little exploration of the seven dimensions as suggested in the family health model has occurred.

A useful consideration would be comparing the seven dimensions of family health and the stages of alcoholism recovery. For example, modifying Brown and Lewis's model to accomodate family health could illustrate the point. Family health suffers in the drinking stage. Factors such as economic uncertainty, physical impact on the alcoholic, possible physical ailments from stress in family members, mental anguish, and emotional volatility tend to promote social, spiritual, and cultural isolation. In the transition stage, the family is in damage-control mode corralling the alcoholism; little energy remains to devote to the seven dimensions of family health. In the early recovery stage, family issues are deemphasized and individual healing and growth are pushed. Some initial stability can lead to incidental family health improvement on some of the seven dimensions, but family health is a low priority. Only in the final stage, ongoing recovery, is there emphasis on family growth. But little discussion occurs of how the seven dimensions of family health are nurtured or how holistic well-being in the family is achieved. Once alcoholism recovery is achieved, the family gets healthier as a composite of individual growth and maturity. Family health seems more a combination of individual family member wellness than an entity that needs nurturing as a gestalt. Support groups in substance abuse—Al-Anon, Alateen, Al-Atot, Alcoholics Anonymous (AA)—are all focused on individual-based recovery. Where is Alcoholic Families Anonymous?

This author proposes that utilizing family health social work practice would be very useful and tie in nicely as part of the transition into Brown and Lewis's ongoing recovery stage, or Jackson's recovery and reunion stage, or Curtis's late recovery stage, or Steinglass's late phase, or Treadway's intimacy stage, or Schlesinger's thriving as a family stage. Regardless of the model, a real need exists to attend to the seven dimensions as families refocus on functioning as a family and seeking holistic well-being. Figure 9.1 shows how the blending of Brown and Lewis's stages and family health model might look.

The primary illustration in Figure 9.1 is the increasing emphasis on family health as an issue of increasing importance in the ongoing recovery stage. Unlike Brown and Lewis's model, the family health model would put a higher effort on facilitating family health than on specific individual recovery efforts. In other words, family health is more than a by-product of individual commitment to recovery. Family well-being must be nurtured and the seven dimensions prioritized as stabilization of alcoholism issues occurs.

## *SIMULATED CASE STUDY*

One way to illustrate the blending of alcoholism family recovery and family health is by means of a case study. Tom Harris is a forty-two-year-old computer repair technician who has been married for fifteen years to forty-year-old Betty, a real estate broker. They have two children, Fred, age thirteen, and Katherine, age twelve. Tom be-

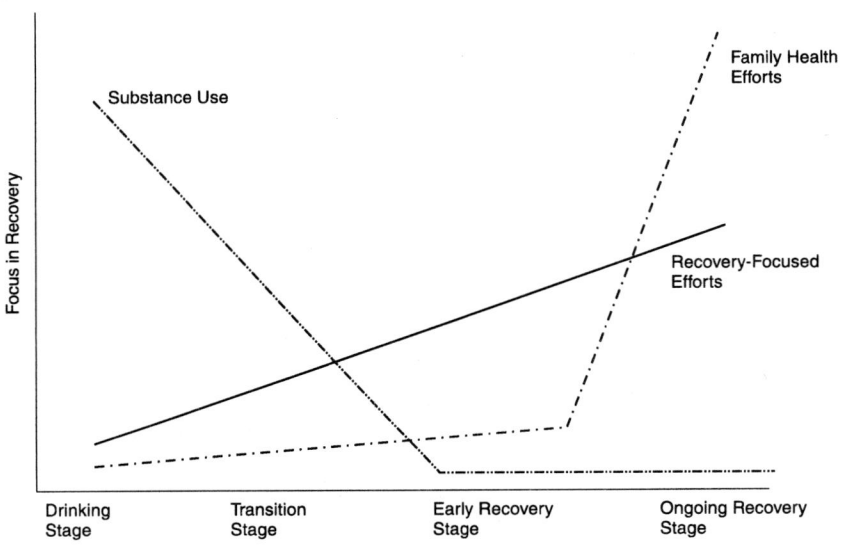

FIGURE 9.1. Illustration of the Combination of the Brown and Lewis Family Recovery Model and Family Health Model

gan drinking heavily ten years ago, with periodic blackouts and verbal explosions at home beginning nine years ago. His spouse initially confronted him about his drinking, but his denial and redirection of the concern into criticizing her led Betty to slowly withdraw from the marriage. Betty noticed Tom's episodes of passing out on the living-room floor, his increasing frequency of staying out all night, and his lack of concern about any family issues or important events, such as birthdays or holidays.

Betty felt increasingly trapped by Tom's drinking. Tom continued to function at work but had retracted from almost all meaningful contact with his family, friends, and extended family. Embarrassed and confused, Betty tried to raise her children as if she were a single parent. Tom's drinking prompted financial difficulties and periodic legal expenses due to his three driving-under-influence (DUI) arrests. Betty sought church support but never revealed Tom's alcoholism. Betty suffered from frequent headaches and chronic fatigue. Five years ago, Tom's fourth DUI forced him into mandated treatment. Betty attended the weekly family session at the outpatient treatment program and began to get support from Al-Anon and assistance from other spouses of alcoholics. When Tom came home, Betty vented her anger at his behavior and gave him an ultimatum: stay sober or leave. Tom struggled and relapsed a few times. Betty stormed and pointed out his failure. Slowly, Tom began to stay sober for longer periods, became a regular AA member, and began working on his recovery. As he committed to staying sober and healing his relationship with his family, Tom was surprised at their resistance. His children were hesitant, even scared at times, when he sought to do activities with them. Betty began to deteriorate and struggled with clinical depression as Tom improved. Fortunately, Tom received regularly scheduled therapy and continued AA support. Betty worked through her depression with a therapist. The couple began working together on undoing the damage to the marriage. Within two years of his completing his mandated treatment, Tom and Betty began to trust and enjoy their relationship. The children slowly began to reembrace the family activities. Their finances have been improving; they have begun socializing with friends and extended family again. In the past year, Betty and Tom have served as AA and Al-Anon sponsors and have successfully completed a marriage enrichment workshop. Tom has begun attending church services with the family and feels that the family is stronger than ever. The children are academically and socially blossoming. Betty finally feels confident that the family will survive Tom's alcoholism.

## FUTURE DIRECTIONS FOR FAMILY HEALTH SOCIAL WORK PRACTICE WITH FAMILIES WITH ALCOHOL ABUSE

The proposed adaptation of the FHSWP model with alcohol-abusing families has significant potential for further exploring how families navigate alcohol abuse issues. However, no empirical validation of the FHSWP model has occurred and the primary direction needs to be basic research confirming the seven dimensions of family health, ways to measure progression toward well-being in each dimension, and verification that the seven dimensions are interconnected and vital to family well-being. Once this basic research is concluded, further research can be conducted on applications of FHSWP to various issues including alcohol abuse. Until that research is concluded, the FHSWP model, similar to other models related to families with alcohol abuse, is just a conceptual supposition based on theoretical and anecdotal beliefs. All theory begins with suppositions. Empirical research validates and refines the suppositions and solidifies the concepts. The Brown and Lewis model has some initial research and hopefully is continuing the research agenda to clarify alcoholism family recovery. Blending the family health model and Brown and Lewis model is a logical extension of the recovery strategies for families with alcoholics.

The theoretical and empirical directions for the FHSWP model strive to offer additional resources for families struggling with the impact of alcohol-abusing family members. Just as a map is not the same as actual terrain, family recovery models seek to summarize the complexities of family issues but are never perfect predictors of reality. Further research will help link that reality with the best models, and much work remains to be accomplished.

## REFERENCES

Brown, S. and Lewis, V. (1995). The alcoholic family: A developmental model of recovery. In S. Brown (Ed.), *Treating alcoholism* (pp. 179-315). San Francisco: Jossey-Bass.

Brown, S. and Lewis, V. (1999). *The alcoholic family in recovery: A developmental model*. New York: Guilford Press.

Cole, E.S. (1995). Becoming family centered: Child welfare's challenge. *Families in Society, 76*(3), 163-172.

Collins, R.L., Leonard, K.E., Searles, J.S. (Eds.) (1990). *Alcohol and the family: Research and clinical perspectives*. New York: Guilford Press.

Comer, E.W. and Fraser, M.W. (1998). Evaluation of six family support programs: Are they effective? *Families in Society 79*(2), 134-148.

Curtis, O. (1999). *Chemical dependency: A family affair*. Pacific Grove, CA: Brooks/Cole.

Denby, R.W., Curtis, C.M., and Alford, K.A. (1998). Family preservation services and special populations: The invisible target. *Families in Society, 79*(1), 3-14.

Duncan, S.F. and Brown, G. (1992). RENEW: A program for building remarried family strengths. *Families in Society, 73*(3), 149-158.

Faria, G. (1994). Training for family preservation practice with lesbian families. *Families in Society, 75*(7), 416-422.

Freeman, E.M. (1993). *Substance abuse treatment: A family systems perspective.* Newbury Park, CA: Sage Publications.

Gorski, T.T. and Miller, M. (1986). *Counseling for relapse prevention.* Independence, MO: Herald House-Independent Press.

Hartman, A. and Laird, J. (1983). *Family-centered social work practice.* New York: The Free Press.

Jackson, J.K. (1954). The adjustment of the family to the crisis of alcoholism. *Quarterly Journal of Studies on Alcohol, 15,* 562-586.

Kelley, P. (1996). Family-centered practice with stepfamilies. *Families in Society, 79*(9), 535-544.

Laird, J. (1995). Family-centered practice in the postmodern era. *Families in Society, 76*(3), 150-162.

Lightburn, A. and Kemp, S.P. (1994). Family support programs: Opportunities for community-based practice. *Families in Society, 75*(1), 16-26.

Munson, C.E. (Ed.) (1980). *Social work with families: Theory and practice.* New York: The Free Press.

Nowinski, J.K. (1999). *Family recovery and substance abuse: A twelve-step guide for treatment.* Thousand Oaks, CA: Sage Publications.

Pardeck, J.T. and Yuen, F.K.O. (1997). A family health approach to social work practice. *Family Therapy, 24,* 115-128.

Pardeck, J.T. and Yuen, F.K.O. (Eds.) (1999). *Family health: A holistic approach to social work practice.* Westport, CT: Auburn House.

Pardeck, J.T., Yuen, F.K.O., Daley, J.G., and Hawkins, C.L. (1998). Social work assessment and intervention through family health practice. *Family Therapy, 25*(1), 25-39.

Pecora, P.J., Fraser, M.W., Nelson, K.E., McCroskey, J. and Meezan, W. (1995). *Evaluating family based services.* New York: Aldine De Gruyter.

Pinderhughes, E. (1995). Empowering diverse populations: Family practice in the 21st century. *Families in Society,* 131-140.

Powell, J.Y. (1996). A schema for family-centered practice. *Families in Society, 77*(7), 446-448.

Reid, W.J. (1985). *Family problem solving.* New York: Columbia University Press.

Rivers, P.C. (1994). *Alcohol and human behavior: Theory, research, and practice.* Englewood Cliffs, NJ: Prentice-Hall

Ronnau, J.P. and Marlow, C.R. (1993). Family preservation, poverty, and the value of diversity. *Families in Society, 74*(9), 538-544.

Rosenberg, H. (1981-1982). Holistic therapy with alcoholism families. *Alcohol, Health, and Research World, 6,* 30-32.

Schlesinger, S.E. and Horberg, L.K. (1994). The "taking charge" model of recovery for addictive families. In J.A. Lewis (Ed.), *Addictions: Concepts and strategies for treatment* (pp. 233-252). Gaithersburg, MD: Aspen Publications.

Seilhamer, R.A. (1991). Effects of addiction on the family. In D.C. Daley and M.S. Raskin (Eds.), *Treating the chemically dependent and their families* (pp. 172-194). Newbury Park, CA: Sage Publications.

Steinglass (1987). *The alcoholic family.* New York: Basic Books.

Sviridoff, M. and Ryan, W. (1997). Community-centered family service. *Families in Society, 78*(2), 128-139.

Treadway (1989). *Before it's too late: Working with substance abuse in the family.* New York: W.W. Norton, Inc.

Vosler, N.R. (1996). *New approaches to family practice: Confronting economic stress.* Thousand Oaks, CA: Sage.

Weick, A. (1986). The philosophical context of a health model of social work. *Social Casework,* 551-559.

Weick, A. and Saleebey, D. (1995). Supporting family strengths: Orienting policy and practice toward the 21st century. *Families in Society, 76*(3), 141-149.

Wells, K. and Beigel, D.E. (Eds.) (1991). *Family preservation services: Research and evaluation.* Newbury Park, CA: Sage.

Werrbach, G.B. (1996). Family strengths-based intensive child case management. *Families in Society,* 216-226.

Yuen, F.K. and Pardeck, J.T. (1999). A family health approach to social work practice. In J.T. Pardeck and F.K. Yuen (Eds.), *Family health: A holistic approach to social work practice* (pp. 1-16). Westport, CT: Auburn House.

Chapter 10

# Family Health Practice with the Spiritually Diverse Person

Francis K. O. Yuen
Doman Lum

## INTRODUCTION

Family health social work practice views spirituality as an integral and important part of one's well-being. Raines (1997) cites Cabot (1927), who defined spiritual diagnosis as the attempt to view the person's central purpose and how one relates to the total parts of the world. Raines also quotes Batson and Ventis's (1982) discussion of spiritual maturity as "an increased tolerance for ambiguity" (1997, p. 8). Joseph (1997) views spirituality as

> a drive, need, power or capacity.... It is that non-material, mysterious aspect of the person, the ground of one's being that strives for meaning, union with universe, and all things.... It seeks to transcend the self, to discover meaning and purpose in the world. It is expressed in form—in the connectedness with nature, in personality, in culture—in the experience of the aesthetic, and in religion or in any form that seeks relatedness to the infinite. (p. 2)

The terms spirituality, faith, and religion are often treated interchangeably. However, each is a distinct term. *Spirituality* is "an inner sense of connectedness and meaningfulness in life" (Raines, 1997, p. 8). *Faith* is "an inner system of beliefs which relate one to the transcendent or ultimate reality, for the theistic believer, God" (Joseph, 1997, p. 2). Conversely, *religion* is "the organized, outward expression of that connection and meaning" (Raines, 1997, p. 8) or "the external expression of one's faith" (Joseph, 1997, p. 2). A good possibility exists that someone can be very spiritual but have no affiliation with any religious organizations. Equally, a very religious individual may not be spiritual.

Raines (1997) develops the typology between spirituality and religiousness into four quadrants. He identifies these types as those who could be (1) religious but not spiritual (means orientation), while some are (2) religious and spiritual (end orientation), (3) neither spiritual nor religious (secular orientation), or (4) spiritual and not religious (quest orientation). People who are extrinsically motivated would use religion as a means to achieve status, power, money, or whatever suits their own ends. Then, some intrinsically motivated people believe and embrace a religion and its creeds for an end by itself. Although some secular people are skeptical about religion and spirituality, others are more open-minded to dialogues and quests for a better understanding of the complexity and tentativeness of the existential questions of life. An example of quadrant 1 is a person who goes to church and observes the rituals of religion but does not have a personal application of faith to daily life. A quadrant 2 individual is a person who has a personal faith and is active in a religious community. A quadrant 3 individual is a person totally devoid of religion and spirituality with a secular and humanistic outlook on life. Finally, a quadrant 4 person has a deep sense of meaning and existence, communes with God and nature, but does not affiliate with an organized religious group.

Family health practice emphasizes the interrelatedness and reciprocal effects of the different aspects of clients' lives. Spiritual well-being is one of these important aspects. It serves as the guiding force and source of meaning for people's lives. Spirituality and spiritual practices are both universal and culturally bounded. Different cultural or ethnic groups have common as well as distinctive outlooks and practices of their spirituality. Family health practice values cultural and spiritual diversity, viewing them as particularly essential when dealing with people of minority backgrounds and experiences, for example, refugees and immigrants.

Refugees and new immigrants often find themselves encountering unfamiliar and stressful environments that demand constant adjustment and coping. Sadly, the most common stable and reliable sources of support, such as family or neighborhood, are no long available or, in some cases, are invalid in the new land. These situations of imbalance and instability between output (e.g., social adjustment and coping) and input (i.e., family or cultural support) exacerbate the difficulties of resettlement. A need for support and a strong desire for stability and equilibrium occurs.

In new environments, people assess and take actions to locate their own new places (niches) that, in turn, affect their interrelatedness with others in the ecosystems. Adjusting to new social and cultural environments involves many major challenges and new life paths. These demands often make people take stock, look inward, and quest transcendentally to attribute meaning to their new existence.

In the face of shifting environments and uncertainties and without the benefits of reliable family and cultural supports, people turn to spirituality and often, operationally, to religion for anchoring and continuity. In place of families and kinships, organized religions have become the support system for many new arrivals and ethnic minority groups. Ethnic-specific religious groups are particularly active in substantiating this role. Unlike ethnic quarters of a city such as Chinatown, Little Italy, or other small-scale ethnic organizations, ethnic religious groups attend to more than social and cultural needs. They help fill the spiritual vacuum and the search for meaning of existence in a new land. Jewish synagogues, Muslim mosques, Asian Buddhist and Taoist temples, African-American Christian churches, and many others serve these vital functions.

In the search for spiritual enlightenment, many have ventured into the spiritual world or religions that are nontraditional to their ethnic or cultural backgrounds. Judaism, Buddhism, and Islamic faiths, to name a few, have gained new followers with diverse backgrounds. It would not be a surprise, for example, to meet someone who is both a Jew and is a practicing Buddhist. The outreach or evangelization efforts of some of these religious groups, however, have not had the same history and aggressiveness as many of the Christian churches.

The Christian churches have a steady history of sending missionaries overseas to evangelize and spread their faiths. Consequently, many of the new arrivals in the United States are familiar with or already are members of a particular Christian faith. During the past several decades, Christian churches have been significant partners in the resettlement of refugees by providing much-needed social services or by sponsoring refugee families. With the increase of the immigrant populations in the United States in the past several decades, many Christian churches have begun to focus on domestic evangelization work with these new arrivals. All of these efforts have brought about increased cultural diversity among some of the Christian churches. Along with the growth of other non-Christian faiths and the popularity of "new age" quests for spiritual enlightenment, the United States has witnessed an increase in people who are both culturally and spiritually diverse.

## THE SPIRITUALLY DIVERSE PERSON

The spiritually diverse person is influenced by spiritual principles and practices and is a member of a community that may or may not be involved with a religious group. A recent text, *Explorations in Counseling and Spirituality: Philosophical, Practical, and Personal Reflections* (Faiver et al., 2001), asserts that spirituality is connected with cultural differences and channeled through and shaped by culture. Among the themes mentioned are the concepts of evil and counseling, human suffering, guilt and mental health, the spirituality of the twelve-step program, and counselor belief system.

Spirituality and cultural diversity are two major variables in the development of the critical consciousness of the spiritually directed person. Reed and colleagues (1997, pp. 46-47) introduce the concept of critical consciousness:

> Critical consciousness incorporates and gives us a greater understanding of power relationships and commonalities and differences among and within people. People create multiple identities based on their life experiences that are shaped by these forces. We need to work to understand people through *their* construction and enactment of their multiple identities. That is, people must be understood in terms of the social/political/historical macro forces influencing their lives and the meaning they as individuals make of these forces. We can also apply our critical skills to understand the social environments around us—our families, organizations, communities, and governments.

Similarities among people as well as differences that foster uniqueness assist us in sorting out our multiple identities and establishing our positions as individuals in relation to others. Reed and associates (1997) further explain the characteristics of positionality:

- An inward process of self-examination and self-exploration and an outward process of understanding and situating oneself in the world
- A dialogue between thinking and action, knowledge and experience, whereby critical reflection and engagement are joined which leads to involvement and commitment
- A newly established position involving a different standpoint from which one develops a level of awareness about one's social location
- A connection between a particular point in your journey through life (positionality) and your perspectives and observations about society (worldview)

Cultural diversity and spirituality are two powerful forces that define one's existential identity and being. These two positions shape the inner being of a person in terms of historical heritage and belief systems, which impacts current and future cognitive perception, affective feelings, and behavioral responses.

In the various major cultural and spiritual people-of-color communities, a range of spirituality occurs that is central to an understanding of cultural groups, especially related to family health practice. Spirituality is at the heart of Native American cultural practices. Indigenous religious rituals and beliefs in the healing power of nature have been maintained through generations to the present in traditional families and tribes. Natural forces are associated with the life process itself and pervade everything the believing Native American does. Community religious rites are a collective effort that promotes nature and increases inward insight and experiential connection with nature. In family health practice, Native Americans can use the positive experiences that result from ceremonial events, power-revealing events (omens, dreams, visions), and contact with a tribal medicinal healer. In working with Native Americans, family health practitioners must learn to explore, understand, and reinforce the therapeutic significance of religious and cultural events (Lewis, 1977).

Spiritual expressions of faith are incorporated in the African-American church and are declared in terms of individual and group singing and clapping of hands, fervent preaching, and responses from worshipers. Religious belief in the deliverance and protection of God was an integral part of the lives of the African slaves who turned to religion to survive the hardships of slavery, prejudice, and racism that they sustained. The African-American Christian church has given credibility to cultural heritage, validated the worth of African Americans, and provided hope for the future. The African-American churches remain a strong moral, educational, and political force speaking out for civil rights, political justice, cultural rediscovery, and family stability and restoration. African-American Protestant theology has articulated a liberation message, analyzing the sins of society in terms of oppression, and proclaiming the good news of liberation and freedom in Christ. This has empowered the church and church members in their struggles.

Likewise, the church has influenced Latino families as a moral force that shapes the ethical behavior of family members. This promotes a spiritual influence on religious instruction, ethnic and cultural holidays and celebrations, and religious practices involving the local ethnic community. In the Catholic Church the priest participates in the life of the Latino community through religious observances and festivals, confirmations, and social services. Catholic Social Services (CSS) maintains an extensive Latino family care program and identifies with the local barrio churches. In many Latino communities CSS sponsors emergency financial aid, home visitation, care for the ill and the elderly, newcomer services, housing, and employment services. The Pentecostal Latino church also promotes a personal, compassionate, evangelical message, as well as provides practical services to meet the needs of Latino families.

Asian Americans attend a variety of religious groups ranging from Buddhist, Protestant, and Catholic congregations that are solely ethnic and cultural in beliefs and practices to Asian Americans integrated into Protestant and Catholic churches with other ethnic groups. Ethnic group churches emphasize strong religious reverence coupled with cultural values and practices such as respect for ancestors and the elders, filial piety, patience, politeness, and avoidance of shame. These moral principles are practiced in the religious and ethnic communities and assist many Asian-American families in their social functioning by defining their obligation, duty, and loyalty to others. Good performance and achievement in school, employment, and community bring honor to the family. Shame and dishonor are powerful motivators to minimize unacceptable behavior. Mental illness and retardation, criminal behavior, job failure, and even poor school grades are kept within the family. To share negative information outside the home is to bring disgrace to the family name. This standard of morality may seem harsh and rigid to outsiders, but to many Asian Americans it helps to maintain order, honor, and harmony in the family.

The interconnection and linkage among personal and corporate spiritual beliefs and practices and ethnic group cultural expressions are to be examined against this background. However, a particular ethnic person with a unique expression of spiritual diversity may chart a different and dissimilar pattern, depending on the situation involved. Never be surprised to discover ethnic and spiritually diverse persons outside the general description.

## *CASE STUDY: THE CASE OF ANNIE*

Annie is a fifteen-year-old teenager from Hong Kong. Her parents, who have a small import/export business in Hong Kong, sent Annie to live with relatives in Monterey Park, California. Annie is the oldest of four siblings and has misgivings about leaving her friends in school behind. Her parents want her to graduate from an American high school so she can be admitted to a University of California school. They see this as an excellent opportunity for their daughter to advance her education and future job possibilities. This is also the opportunity for her to establish possible residency and citizenship. Her relatives in California consist of an uncle and aunt in their early forties; they have been married for fifteen years and have two younger children of their own. They moved to the United States from Malaysia about twenty years ago.

After arriving, Annie had initial difficulties adjusting to her new environment for several months. She missed her familiar surroundings in Hong Kong, her family, and most of all her friends in school. She is a *parachute kid* (literally dropped into an American community from an Asian country of origin without family and friends) who is separated from her primary nuclear family and is going through her teenage identity crisis with her surrogate parents, her uncle and aunt.

Annie understands her parents' desires for her to have a better future, a good life. She also is aware that her success may provide the future opportunities for her siblings and her parents to join her in the United States. However, she is uncertain, angry, and frustrated about why she is in the United States. She questions the meaning of such drastic actions. In fact, she doubts the meaning of the so-called "good life" that required the breakup of her family and her own life.

For the most part, Annie is a loner in school. She is afraid of meeting other students; her mediocre abilities in English make her feel insecure and incompetent. She was an A student in Hong Kong, but her academic performance in her American school is just below C. She is disappointed in herself and is emotionally rather miserable. Annie feels the need to fulfill her family obligations to do well in school; she also blames herself and her parents for getting her in such a situation. Several times in the past month, she found herself not able to get up from bed in the morning to go to school. She has lost interest in everything, including school and her favorite pastime of e-mailing her friends back in Hong Kong.

Annie complains about physical symptoms such as headache, muscle cramps, fatigue, and an overwhelming feeling of sickness. In her correspondence with her parents and in conversations with one of the female students from Hong Kong in her school, she has made comments to the effect that she does not care anymore whether she lives or dies. Both her aunt and her schoolteacher became aware of her situation through Annie's parents and the other Hong Kong student. Her aunt and schoolteacher met and decided to refer Annie to the school social worker, Ms. Freeman.

In preparation for Annie, Ms. Freeman met with a Chinese-American teacher at the school to gain better understanding of cultural and other issues related to students from Hong Kong. She "came across" Annie on campus and asked if Annie minded choosing a place in the school where they could talk. Annie was reluctant to meet with Ms. Freeman at first, although she appreciated and enjoyed the attention. During the first few individual sessions, Ms. Freeman was able to develop the trust and rapport that allowed Annie to discuss her problems. Annie wants to be sure that confidentiality will be maintained and that her parents and relatives are not going to know all the details of what they discuss. Ms. Freeman agrees; however, she also emphasizes that, with Annie's agreement, they may need to include her parents or aunt and uncle in future discussions.

In addition to working with the social worker individually on her mental health concerns and with a school tutor on her academic performance, Annie follows Ms. Freeman's recommendations to participate in more outside activities. Reluctantly, she joins the school English Conversation Club, a support group set up by the social worker and an English teacher for nonnative English-speaking students. Annie also tries to join the school choir.

Through the English Conversation Club, Annie meets a friendly new Chinese girl who invites her to attend her youth group at a local Chinese-speaking church. Annie discusses this invitation with her social worker. Ms. Freeman encourages Annie to give it a try, if it does not contradict her personal faith and culture. Ms. Freeman also points out that on quite a few occasions Annie has asked transcendental questions during their meetings. It appears to Ms. Freeman that Annie is searching not only for personal identity but also for purpose and meaning for herself. This might be one possible way for Annie to further her quest. Annie used to go to church in Hong Kong through the Christian school that she attended, but she was not very interested in religion. She also went to the Buddhist and Taoist temples with her parents and relatives. Her family celebrated traditional, cultural, and religious holidays at home including Buddhist and Taoist festivals and ceremonies as well as Christianity's Christmas and Easter.

Despite her lack of interest in religion, Annie finds a sense of togetherness in this new Chinese youth group. Most are American-born Chinese, with a few overseas-born Chinese, like Annie. She is readily accepted by the group and enjoys the weekly meetings and monthly socials. Spiritually, she enjoys discussions on the meaning and purpose of life within the Chinese cultural context with other Chinese. She comes together as a spiritual and a culturally diverse person and finds her identity in this group.

Annie's parents, similar to many Chinese, practice a diffused religion that has a mix of traditional Buddhism and Taoism with many gods. Her uncle and aunt, with their Malaysian background, are practicing Muslims. All of them are familiar with the Christian faith. They recognize the contributions that Christian churches make in the lives of young people and are supportive of their activities. They are relieved at this acculturated adjustment and are thankful to the ethnic religious organizations for making a contribution to the well-being of their daughter and niece. Upon consultations with Annie parents, the aunt and uncle have planned to meet with Ms. Freeman to find ways that can make Annie "a better and happier kid."

## ASSESSMENT AND DIAGNOSTIC IMPRESSIONS

Annie is experiencing cultural and social adjustment difficulties. She is uncertain of how her past relates to her new environment. As a teenager, she is still in the process of establishing her own identity. Instead, she has been charged with the responsibility of not only becoming independent in a foreign land but also paving the way for her family to come to America. Annie has not developed the coping skills to meet her personal needs and her family obligations. She is uncertain about the worthiness and the meaning of such an overseas venture. A sense of emptiness and a lack of purpose pervades, hindering Annie's commitment and motivation to move forward.

As a teen, Annie is forming her own identity. She is struggling with the big question of who she is. Culturally, she is willing to obey her family's grand plan for her. However, personally, she is unsure that this is the best arrangement for her and her future. In fact, the future has been a matter of little concern in her life as a teenager who was enjoying school, friends, and family in Hong Kong. Spiritually, Annie is not religious but has the desire for open dialogue and exploration. She believes her new church connections may be a good way for her to develop a better understanding of the meaning and purpose of life.

Family health practice with diverse populations concerns availability, accessibility, and acculturation (Yuen, 1999). Although Annie has her uncle and aunt's family to turn to, her familiar and reliable support systems such as her immediate family and close friends in Hong Kong are no longer readily available or accessible to her. Many universities and colleges have programs to deal with the special needs of international students. Most high schools are less prepared although willing to meet this demand. It may not be too long until Annie familiarizes herself with American culture and becomes just one of the kids in the school. However, until that time, Annie faces the daunting task of acculturating and developing new understanding of her environment and the associated coping skills.

## PROBLEM SOURCES AND MANIFESTATIONS

Cultural and social adjustment difficulties and lack of support systems appear to be the presenting problems for Annie. Her main source of distress, however, rests more on her sense of lack of meaning for herself and her situation. Culturally, Annie follows through with her obligations as a dutiful daughter and the oldest child to fulfill the family's desire. Personally, Annie was not prepared for the loneliness and alienation that she encountered. Annie had enjoyed a well-functioning and balanced ecosystem in Hong Kong. In place of that, she finds herself in an off-balance and uncertain system; she is having difficulties locating her niche and relating to others. She also does not have adequate coping skills that allow her to deal with the life stresses of being a teenager in a new land.

Annie's difficulties have gone unnoticed for a long period of time, although she exhibited a variety of symptoms of depression and psychosomatic complaints. Even with the change of school environments, her poor school performance represented a drastic change in her usual accomplishments. Her hints of lack of interest in living and her depressive moods are further evidence of her difficulties and her attempts to get help.

## INTERVENTION SKILLS

Culturally competent family health practice includes several major considerations (Yuen, 1999, pp. 108-109):

1. Accessibility, availability, and acculturation
2. Utilization and identification of effective point of entry (for prefessional interventions)
3. Extensive contacts in a client's environment to allow the building of a productive working relationship
4. Family as well as the individual as the units of intervention
5. Culturally appropriate assessment and intervention procedures

Ms. Freeman seeks consultation in the school from a Chinese-American teacher who understands Annie's cultural and social background. Ms. Freeman keeps Annie's identity anonymous, allowing her to be culturally more in tune with Annie. She "came across" Annie on campus and allowed Annie to choose a place where they could meet, thereby giving back the sense of control and safety that Annie needed in her own environment. Ms. Freeman has made herself accessible and available to Annie, with sensitivity to Annie's issues of acculturation. She promotes the environments that are easy for Annie to engage in with the various services that she could provide. Ms. Freeman is working with Annie on personal issues, and she also includes family as the unit of intervention. Specifically, interventions for Annie should consider the following.

1. Annie needs a simple problem-solving/task-centered approach, which identifies her problem of acculturation and transition into a new and different environment. By identifying her needs and issues, appropriate interventions that produce both short-term concrete outcomes as well as long-term results can be developed. Concrete and specific results are particularly useful to decrease Annie's chance of dropping out and to build hope to pursue further services that she needs.

2. Similarly, utilization of social constructionist approaches (e.g., Franklin and Nurius, 1998) and existential orientations (e.g., Harper and Lantz, 1996) can help Annie fill her existential vacuum and assist in her search for meaning in her new life in this new environment.

3. On the mezzolevel, one probable alternative is to help her find a new accepting group that meets her unique needs. Organizations focusing on group purpose, activities, and new member outreach such as social community service programs, religious groups, and ethnic organizations are helpful vehicles for persons in need of adjustment. Annie found the meaning and power in a group that reaches out, accepts her, and gives her a collective identity and personality. This group cushions the loss of family and friends in Hong Kong and gives her a purpose for living and thriving in a new California setting. The church community also provides a new reference group and a new niche for her to anchor and relate to others in the ecosystems.

4. Annie needs to hear a message of acceptance and empowerment, which builds on individual worth, group recognition, and solidarity. Most spiritual and religious services engender such beliefs, confirmed through their rituals and practical acts of love, acceptance, and caring. Annie feels empowered by this group of new friends who are absorbing her into their world and their activities. Annie experi-

ences such existential qualities of personal self-worth, self-actualization, unconditional acceptance, empathy for her situation, being and becoming, and human purpose and functioning. These concepts are embodied in her experiences with her new friends.

5. Involving Annie's families at the appropriate time to gain their support and understanding of Annie's needs and concerns is essential to build clinical alliance to further Annie's causes within her family and cultural contexts.

6. The religious organization forms a natural alliance for refugees and immigrants who are in the process of resettlement as well as for any newcomer to a strange community. Many religious organizations provide an instant group of friends, a slate of weekly activities, social and employment contacts, and related opportunities for adjustment. Family health social workers should also educate themselves to become knowledgeable enough to distinguish spiritual concerns from religious ones, and cult organizations from bona fide religious or spiritual ones. Social workers utilize organizations, including religious ones, to meet clients' spiritual and other needs. At the same time, they should maintain their professional objectivity and not becoming proselytizers for religious organizations within their practice.

7. In working with Annie on spirituality-related issues, a family health social worker should be cognizant of several areas of concerns on cultural and spiritual practice:

    a. *Spousal relationships:* Gender roles and expectations differ from culture to culture and in various religious groups. Although some are in tune with liberal views, some embrace more rigid notions. Some fundamental religious groups have a strong sense of moral and theological certainty that affects spousal relationships. A family health social worker should be mindful of the gender and spousal relationships between Annie's parents and between her uncle and aunt. These relationships have strong implications for the dynamics and decision-making process for the family and its dependents.

    b. *Parent/child relationships:* Along with the stronger sense of morality among certain faiths, an increased awareness of human dysfunction, weakness, and limitations occurs with corresponding high disciplinary expectations and practices. Family health social workers need to be conscious of these preferences and work with them within the legal and ethical contexts. The skillful integration and influx of the strength perspectives with Annie and her family can facilitate the attainment of a more balanced focus. Culturally, Asian groups have high expectations of their children to carry on or build family honor. Being the oldest child, Annie would be expected to take on an even more significant role in helping out the family.

  c. *Sexual issues:* Dating, sexual relationships, abortion, homosexuality, and the like are common topics of concern for many teens. Different religious groups have varying degrees of tolerance or acceptance for such issues. It is likely that Annie's spiritually diverse backgrounds and her Hong Kong Chinese cultural upbringing may not support her in addressing these sexual issues until she finishes her formal education. That Annie did not mention dating or other sexual issues in her meetings with Ms. Freeman may or may not imply that these issues are currently part of her concerns. These are, however, sensitive issues that should be part of the ongoing assessment.

A family health social worker can expect many challenges in working with a spiritually diverse person. Among the challenges are: maintaining an open-minded and meaningful dialogue with clients on sensitive issues that involve personal convictions; getting to know the client's spiritual journey well and close enough to provide support; and remaining distant enough to promote growth without interference.

## *EVALUATION*

An intervention plan or agreement for Annie should first be established with clear objectives to be achieved. These objectives should cover concerns regarding Annie's mental health condition, that is, depression; her cultural and social adjustment issues; connections with supportive organizations; and spiritual needs. Through process recording and documentation of Annie's self-report, Annie's progress will be monitored. Pre- and postintervention assessments using established depression, acculturation, and other appropriate scales will be necessary to evaluate the effectiveness of the interventions. Meanwhile, the cultural competency of these scales, and therefore their validity, should be first critically evaluated to assess their appropriateness.

Spiritual growth is a difficult construct to define and to measure in quantifiable terms. A social worker could measure the frequency, intensity, and duration of certain behavioral indicators of Annie's gains in spirituality as detailed in the intervention objectives. Such indicators may include frequency and extent of participation in youth group activities. Qualitative methods such as a reflective report or journal by Annie along with discussions with the social worker will also be good ways to measure her gains. Reports from Annie's teacher, uncle, and aunt will supplement Annie's self-report and the social worker's observation and assessment.

## REFERENCES

Faiver, C., Ingersoll, R. E., O'Brien, E., and McNally, C. (2001). *Explorations in counseling and spirituality: Philosophical, practical, and personal reflections.* Belmont, CA: Wadsworth/Thomson Learning.

Franklin, C. and Nurius, P. (1998). *Constructivism in practice: Methods and challenges.* Milwaukee, WI: Families International.

Harper, K. and Lantz, J. (1996). *Cross-cultural practice social work with diverse populations.* Chicago: Lyceum.

Joseph, M. V. (1997). Toward the future: Call, covenant, mission. *Society for Spirituality and Social Work Newsletter,* 4(1), 1-5, 10-11.

Lewis, R. (1977). Cultural perspective on treatment modalities with Native Americans. Paper presented at the National Association of Social Workers Symposium, San Diego, CA.

Raines, J. (1997). Spiritual assessment: An initial framework. *Society for Spirituality and Social Work Newsletter,* 4(1), 8-9.

Reed, B. G., Newman, P. A., Suarez, Z. E., and Lewis, E. A. (1997). Interpersonal practice beyond diversity and toward social justice: The importance of critical consciousness. In C. D. Garvin and B. A. Seabury (Eds.), *Interpersonal practice in social work: Promoting competence and social justice* (pp. 44-77). Boston: Allyn & Bacon.

Yuen, F. K. O. (1999). Family health and cultural diversity. In J. T. Pardeck and F. K. O. Yuen (Eds.), *Family health: A holistic approach to social work practice* (pp. 101-114). Westport, CT: Auburn House.

Chapter 11

# The Management of a Family Health and Family-Based Services Agency

Francis K. O. Yuen
John Gunther

Pardeck and Yuen (1999) profile family health social work practice as a new model of providing services to families. Family health moves beyond family-centered practice in that it goes beyond family therapy and moves family into an ecosystems perspective. The ecosystems perspective is important because it begins to account for policy dimensions and service delivery systems that empower families and the community context in which they reside. The National Association of Social Workers (NASW) emphasizes the need for this most important consideration. Mayden and Nieves (2000) note:

> Family supports [and agencies] should encompass a comprehensive infrastructure of economic and social entitlement, including health care, income supports, family allowance, access to employment, education, dependent care, housing and social services. Comprehensive services should include a continuum that enhances functioning and prevents dysfunction and intensive intervention to alleviate problems. (p. 120)

## *FAMILY HEALTH AGENCY SERVICES*

For the management and administration of program or agency and at the policy level, family health practice refers to the concerns and supports for the family's involvement in interventions as provided through financing, policies and procedures, staffing, training, record keeping, and the structure and organizations of the program or the agency itself.

Family health practice-oriented management and administration embody the support and focus for families and their involvements in the service delivery system. These concerns are manifested through the actualization of the organizational philosophy and the management of the agency and its programs. Staffing, training, program designs, policy and procedures, record keeping, and evaluations are all parts of the mechanisms through which the family health focus is emphasized.

A family health-based agency focuses its policies, procedures, management, and services on the family unit. Although the agency may utilize a variety of family therapy modalities, these are only part of the product mix, which also consists of networking and community coordination that enhance family functioning. It is a family-based service agency that processes specialized knowledge, skills, and interest to serve the family unit. This is an agency that involves the family as a partner in the decision-making and goal-setting process and uses the family's existing resources. It strives to enhance the family members' sense of control over their own lives. The result is that family members feel an increased sense of competence in conducting their lives and can create a safe and nurturing family environment (Berg, 1994, pp. 1-3).

### *Principles of Organizing a Family Health Agency*

In organizing a family health agency, principles regarding families must guide management in its planning, product and service mix, and community coordination. Product and service mix refer to the array of interventions available to families in terms of programs, community outreach, and service interventions. Such a mix might include programs such as parenting classes, advocacy, and family therapy. The following are some of these family-focused principles.

1. The family is at the center of all services.
2. The family should be broadly defined so as to be inclusive.
3. Planning and implementation of service delivery should consider the social policies that affect families and the community context in which the families exist.

4. Practitioners must be trained both in breadth and in depth, focusing on issues impacting today's families. These issues include: poverty, domestic violence, substance and sexual abuse, child welfare and adoption, physical and mental health, older adult care, and child care.
5. The agency, its staff, management, and services must be accountable to the family, the community, and the profession.

## BUILDING A FAMILY HEALTH AGENCY VERSUS A FAMILY SERVICE AGENCY

Some contend that a family health approach to agency building is redundant and mirrors the family service agencies that already exist. Although similarities between the two approaches exist, significant differences are also present. This section delineates the differences between the two approaches in terms of strategic planning, community resource coordination, political advocacy, board development and operations, and management approaches and skills.

### *Strategic Planning*

Strategic planning is "a disciplined effort to produce fundamental decisions and actions that shape and guide what an organization is, what it does, and why it does it" (Bryson and Alston, 1996, pp. 4-5). It is not a static event. It is "an on-going process, reflected in strategic management: strategic thinking and strategic acting" (Lewis et al., 2001, p. 47).

Strategic planning in human service agencies is directed toward the opportunities and threats that exist in an agency's community context. An important consideration in the strategic planning process is to differentiate an agency's product mix from other delivery systems. In terms of differentiation, current family service agencies are primarily characterized by a focus on children living in the family context, family therapy, individual counseling, and family life education. Although these functions are important, they clearly do not sufficiently include community, political, and policy context of family well-being. Svirdoff and Ryan (1997) validate these pehnomena. They observe that although distressed families encounter multiple interrelated problems (e.g., homelessness, poverty, crime, high-risk behaviors, and school and education), most family service agencies only offer family counseling services. Community building oriented interventions represent a very small portion of their services.

In contrast, family health agencies strategically extend themselves beyond counseling into community building and coordination, including family-related policy advocacy and networking. They commit their energy and resources to focus on supporting programming in the community. They recognize the various forms of diversities in the community and develop cultural competency in services. In this matter, both the family and the service provided are grounded in an environment of hope for the improvement of the families in the community.

## *Resource Coordination*

Resources in a typical family service agency are primarily directed toward finding personnel and finances targeting family therapy and primary prevention activities. Resources in a family health agency are designed to give direct access to families living within a neighborhood context. Further, in a family health agency, resources are directed toward activities that not only localize the integration of services but also develop advocacy networks of families that are empowered to overcome the negative valuations and contexts in which families live.

A good example of such orientation is the patch-based community services. This community-centered service delivery approach developed in Britain has shown promising results in its use in Iowa and Pennsylvania (Adams and Krauth, 1995). Each limited geographical area (patch) is serviced by a team of local human service providers. These localized workers operate with different levels and types of skills and functions in the neighborhood offices; they are familiar with the local cultural and physical environments. They also develop formal and informal partnerships within their patches or neighborhoods. Their neighborhood offices enable patch teams to "offer accessible, flexible, and holistic services.... The team is a central element of the patch approach that enables the sharing of knowledge and expertise. Although a team may include several specialists, it is still able to provide a generalist, holistic service" (p. 87).

## Political Advocacy

In this new millennium, families and communities continue to be plagued by the problems of poverty, violence, abuse, and the lack of proper care for vulnerable populations. If the family is to survive, the holistic approach to service delivery is needed, so that services can respond properly to the multiple problems faced by families. Although family therapy services will still be highly valued and needed, service providers recognize that substantive refocusing of services must occur in family-related social policies which are ultimately strengthening families. This focus demands political advocacy. Political advocacy in the eyes of family health agencies is conceived of as a process of empowerment that is initiated by raising the critical consciousness and action taken by families in the community. Families in the community develop a critical consciousness of the problems that exist in their community context. They then meet in groups and empower themselves with legislative representatives to overcome the various identified barriers. They examine the oppressive and discriminatory aspects of these problems. Of course, both legislators and families are constantly coordinating their work with family-oriented agencies in the community. In this regard Hardcastle, Wencour, and Powers (1997, p. 252) have laid down some excellent rules of practice for working the system. They suggest:

1. Learn the decision-making process in the agency and for the particular course of action in which you are interested.
2. Learn who has formal authority for making decisions, as well as who has informal influence with decision makers and in the organization or department generally.
3. Build your social capital in the organization by developing positive exchange relationships with other members of the organization and with organizational decision makers.
4. Build your social capital by establishing your expertise and competence to manage a particular problem area.
5. Learn as much as you can about the rules that will be bent or avoided by your course of action.
6. Search for loopholes, contradictory rules, or cases in which exceptions were made previously as support for your action.

7. Decide whether your course of action requires a formal decision or whether you are better off exercising personal discretion or handling the matter informally.
8. Use the informal system to get necessary information and compare notes.
9. If necessary, draw on your social capital to accomplish your objectives.

## *Board Development and Operations*

Accountability and outcome-based program planning have been the focuses for human services for many years. Yet as the American Humane Association (AHA, 2000, p. 1) has pointed out:

> The overwhelming majority of public and private agencies facing these challenges have difficulty articulating a clear list of qualitative outcomes and benchmarks for which their organizations are accountable. At the same time, funders . . . are demanding that organizations determine what outcomes will be achieved with funds provided and that evidence of this achievement be demonstrated on a regular basis. . . . If an organization, its board, and executive director themselves are not clear about what "success" means, it is quite unlikely anyone else (the community, funders, or the media) will think that the organization is providing value.

Given the current results-oriented environment, it is incumbent on boards of directors of family health agencies to transform their roles. They should go beyond the basic functions such as setting the agency directions and oversight of the executive director on the implementation and actualization of the agency's goals. More attention needs to be focused on strategic leadership. Board members must become more active in setting agency goals, defining board of directors' and the agency staff's boundaries, monitoring the executive director's performance, assuring the sufficiency of resources, and working positively with key organizational stakeholders. This should be an active board that has its own recruitment, development, and organizational plans that produce results. All these activities should result in the strengthening of the foundation and framework of the agency in its services to promote the well-being of families.

## Management Approaches and Skills

Organizational management theories and approaches have gone through many changes that largely correlate to the social and cultural environments at the time. These approaches have evolved from the early discussions on bureaucracy and scientific management to the human relation approach; theory X and theory Y (decision-making power between management and workers); organizational culture; and the recent search for excellence, reinvention, and management of diversity. Depending on the needs and maturity of the organization, the board of directors, executive director, and other management staff should explore and develop their appropriate, while possibly diverse, management approaches. Ideally, these management approaches complement each other and would ultimately bring about positive impacts to the families being served.

## CASE STUDY

The Association for the Betterment of Community (ABC) was established in 1970 to address the special needs of ethnic populations, particularly refugees in California. From its beginning until the early 1990s, it mainly was a mental health outpatient agency. Paraprofessional mental health counselors from various ethnic backgrounds staffed the agency. Licensed clinical social workers and psychologists supervised these counselors. Part-time contracts with various local psychiatrists supported its medication clinic. Financially, it survived mostly on county-contracted funding and Medi-Cal reimbursements. The agency had been meeting unique service needs and was able to secure basic service contracts. ABC provided much-needed culturally relevant mental health services to its clients. Similarly, they also helped the local county mental health department in fulfilling its responsibility to provide culturally appropriate services to newly arrived refugees.

As an outpatient mental health agency in and of itself this agency had a fine program that drew the only available funding at the time for service and filled the needed service gaps. Due to the nature of the problems that it addressed, its services involved mostly refugees and their families. This evolved into a family service agency that provided mental health therapy to various members in the family. The service delivery model, however, was still individual based.

As funding was limited in the 1980s and the early 1990s, and upon the realization of the limitations of individual mental health treatment services with refugee families, the agency sought out various types of service programs and funding sources. This was done under the newly hired deputy chief director, who also oversaw the Families and Children Programs. Among the first wave of nonmental health treatment programs were those for domestic violence intervention, school-based intervention, and substance abuse prevention. Local or state funding initially funded all of these programs. These supports were the results of heavy involvement in lobbying and advocacy on the agency's behalf by the members of the newly reorganized board of directors.

A key question to these expansions was the continuing funding support, or the lack of it, for these new programs. Under the guidance of the executive director, the agency helped put together many ethnic-based community organizations. In turn, they formed alliances with the agency to further advocate for attention and funding from the local government agencies. Gradually, the agency and the alliances developed political status within the local power structure. In fact, the agency had become a major power broker, which was evident by the large number of local politicians in the agency's annual fund-raising banquet that also honored local social and political leaders.

Riding on its successes at the local level, the agency reached out to major federal funding to support its newly conceptualized idea of culturally competent and comprehensive service to families. The chief deputy director successfully landed two major federal grants and almost doubled the agency's annual budget. These multimillion-dollar grants went to support a youth substance abuse treatment program and a high-risk behaviors intervention program that included a youth center, school-based intervention programs, parenting, family involvement activities, weekend cultural schools, and community enhancement activities. In addition, other, smaller state and federal funding supported a safe house for refugee women who were victims of domestic violence, a community health center initiative, and other culturally appropriate family-based programs. All of these new activities aimed to improve the functioning of the target refugee families, their members, and the communities in which they reside. They also augmented the much-needed mental health treatment program.

Increasingly, staff development activities were scheduled to focus on the development and application of a multilevel and multimethod intervention approach to address problems faced by refugee families. Also, for the first time, client representatives were invited to join the board of directors. Its use of professional and paraprofessional staff from the different ethnic groups that the agency served helped to ensure the cultural relevancy and competence of the agency's services.

As the agency shifted from a mental health agency to a family-health-oriented community agency, newly discovered problems regarding the inappropriate use of funding started to surface. Subsequent financial and service audits revealed that apparently funds were embezzled by the executive director and clients' charts were altered by the administrative staff, that is, secretaries, to incur extra Medi-Cal funding. In addition, the audits revealed the unethical and unspoken agency policy of repeatedly changing clients' diagnoses to get more Medi-Cal money and to meet the county service contract requirements.

Led by a group of midlevel managers including the chief deputy director, a two-year "revolution" to reclaim justice, ethical practice, and service to the families in the communities took place. These efforts triggered several investigations by different funding sources. Findings of investigations resulted in the transfer of several major fundings and programs to a similar agency in the community, the replacement of the executive director, selection of a new board of directors with more oversight authority, and stronger demands for accountability within the agency.

## ASSESSMENT AND DIAGNOSTIC IMPRESSIONS

This is a case of agency in transition into a family-health-focused agency. This is also a case of management and mismanagement, ethical practice, cultural competency, roles and responsibilities of board of directors, and self-advocacy among staff and on behalf of clients. Individual greediness, organizational culture, improvement of service mix, and ultimately rapid agency growth provide the backdrop and challenge for managing an agency in transition.

Family health agency management applies all basic management skills and knowledge with a special focus on how the changes affect the agency's nature.

## SOURCE OF THE PROBLEM AND MANIFESTATIONS

As the agency moved from a mental health-based family service agency to a more family health-oriented agency, power and money attracted the top administrator and a situation of "goal displacement" took place. Originally, the agency existed to serve families and their communities. Unfortunately, at the end, the families and communities were used to serve the purpose of getting more and more funding for the agency and its executive director.

With the shift of attention from solely mental health to a more comprehensive family health agency, the agency produced a more desirable service mix to serve the various needs of the refugee communities and families more efficiently. It is also becoming more of a community agency than a specialty one. Consistent with growth and the more holistic orientation, the agency needs to revisit and update its organizational culture and structure; the balance between growth and focus; and, most important, its missions and accountability to its constituencies.

## INTERVENTION STRATEGIES

The agency should develop a rolling strategic plan that includes a service mix that addresses the multiple needs of the individuals and their families. This service mix will include the basic mental health- and problem-oriented interventions, as well as strength- and resiliency-oriented family and community programs. The rolling strategic plan is a three-year plan with a new third year added on annually.

With leadership from the midlevel managers and participation from the line staff and top administrators, a three-year plan will be developed. All staff in the agency will review and adopt this plan with the understanding that it is a dynamic document that requires ongoing revisions. In the second half of each year, through a committee or other mechanism, the agency and its staff will assess the accomplishments and add the new third year to the plan. Using the SWOT (strength, weakness, opportunity, and threat) analysis, the agency will assess its situations and develop appropriate strategic plans. This strategic planning process will develop specific goals and objectives to be achieved during each of the years.

As resource mismanagement was a major problem for the agency, carefully developed resource allocation procedures and their rationales should be in place to ensure proper allocations of resources. An annual financial audit for the whole agency by an outside accounting firm will no longer be a preferred practice but a mandated activity. Certainly, individual programs will also be audited to meet the specific funding requirements.

To ensure the availability of resources including funding, personnel, facilities, and other resources to meet service needs, the agency should be proactive in securing external funding. This can be done by having a paid or volunteer grant writer who can train and assist top and midlevel managers in preparing service grant and contract applications. Each program should also be informed about budgetary situations and be held accountable for the proper use of these resources to promote family well-being. Collectively, a management team, made up of top and midlevel managers as well as representatives from the line staff, should make recommendations and decisions regarding many aspects of the agency's operation, including resource allocations. Resource allocations should also reflect the family health orientation of the agency they go to support—not only problem-oriented program expenses but also those that promote prevention and family-related policies and activities.

Political advocacy is a form of empowerment. Due to funding and nonprofit status restrictions, this agency should be careful in making sure none of its restricted funding is being used for political purposes. Political advocacy for this agency is similar to social advocacy with the employment of many strategies and tactics of political activities. Advocating on behalf of the underserved, the poor, and the oppressed is part of the social work tradition. The agency has started to organize mutual aids groups for different ethnic communities. With careful nurturing and support, these mutual groups will soon become self-sufficient and have the capacity to operate on their own. Meanwhile, the agency can play a convener role in bringing all of them to the table to identify common needs, strategize, and celebrate successes.

The newly restructured board of directors and management reaffirm their commitment to develop a family health-oriented agency. It may take several years to rebuild this agency; however, the prospects are optimistic and the lesson has been learned that family, not the agency and the staff, is the prime focus and goal for the existence of a family health-oriented agency.

The board of directors should become very active and participatory for a limited time to provide technical support and direction for the agency in transition. Hiring a competent executive director will be the board's most urgent task. In the interim, board members as individuals could be politically active in advocating causes that are common with those of the agency. Their connections with the funding sources and their professional expertise in management, funding development, accounting, program development, and particular fields of knowledge will be helpful for the agency in bringing in needed funding and acquiring professional assistance. This active involvement in the day-to-day operation of the agency should be temporary and end after a new director comes on board.

The board should also develop its own recruitment, development, and organizational plan to strengthen the agency and its families. Former service recipients and community members should be part of the board of directors. The board of directors will also take an active role to go out to the community to identify community leaders, professionals, and influential individuals to become potential board members.

Both the top administers and the midlevel program coordinators should spend time to identify and develop managerial skills. Family health agency encourages participation, produces desirable outcomes, and celebrates achievements. Examples of relevant managerial skills and principles include requiring a value-driven and hands-on leadership style; recognizing people (clients, families, and agency staff) as the only asset for the agency; and promoting outcome-based services and performance. The agency also values human diversity, ensures and supports ethnical practice, expands service and agency boundaries, develops productive working relations, uses paraprofessionals effectively, and achieves improved service coordination.

## STRATEGIES TO EVALUATE INTERVENTION

Accompanying the strategic plan is its evaluation plan. With clear program objectives and goals, the agency should be able to assess its abilities in meeting the preset goals and objectives. Since program evaluation is often not considered part of the service structure, it is often overlooked or minimized. To ensure that program evaluation is an integral part of the agency, a director of research and development is recommended. This professional will oversee all the evaluation efforts with support for each of the program staff and also will be responsible for turning over the findings to the top administrators and other relevant individuals to use in decision making.

## REFERENCES

Adams, P. and Krauth, K. (1995). Working with families and communities: The patch approach. In P. Adams and K. Nelson (Eds.), *Reinventing human services* (pp. 87-108). New York: Aldine De Gruyter.

American Humane Association (AHA) (2000). *Child protection leader.* Englewood, CO: Author.

Berg, I. K. (1994). *Family based services: A solution-focused approach.* New York: Norton.

Bryson, J. and Alston, F. (1996). *Creating and implementing your strategic plan.* San Francisco, CA: Jossey-Bass.

Hardcastle, D. A., Wencour, S., and Powers, P. R. (1997). *Community practice.* Oxford, NY: University Press.

Lewis, J., Lewis, M., Packard, T., and Souflée, F. (2001). *Management of human service programs.* Belmont, CA: Brooks/Cole.

Mayden, R. W. and Nieves, J. (2000) *Social work speaks: National Association of Social Workers Policy Statements 2000-2003,* Fifth edition. Washington, DC: NASW Press.

Pardeck, J. T. and Yuen, F. K. O. (1997). A family health approach to social work practice. *Family Therapy, 2*(24), 115-128.

Pardeck, J. T. and Yuen, F. K. O. (1999). *Family health: A holistic approach to social work practice.* Westport, CT: Auburn House.

Svirdoff, M. and Ryan, M. (1997). Community centered family service. *Families in Society: Journal of Contemporary Human Services, 48*(2), 125-139.

Chapter 12

# Americans with Disabilities Act and Family Health

John T. Pardeck

## INTRODUCTION

President George Bush signed the Americans with Disabilities Act (ADA) into law on July 26, 1990. The ADA is viewed as the most progressive civil rights legislation ever enacted in the United States (Pardeck, 1998). The ADA covers both public and private sectors of American life. For example, private businesses have had to make numerous changes in their hiring practices which help to insure that persons with disabilities are not discriminated against in the workplace. Public agencies, including human service agencies, also must make special efforts aimed at preventing discrimination based on disability in the area of social service delivery.

The ADA has five titles that prohibit discrimination against persons with disabilities in the following areas:

1. Employment*
2. Government activities
3. Public services and accommodations
4. Telecommunications
5. Retaliation

---

*In *Board of Trustees of University of Alabama v. Garrett* (99-1240) 193 f.3d 1214, reversed; the United States Supreme Court ruled that state employees are no longer covered by Title I.

In sum, the ADA provides a national mandate designed to eliminate discrimination against persons with disabilities in virtually all aspects of American life.

The ADA is based on two major civil rights laws: (1) the Civil Rights Act of 1964 and (2) the Rehabilitation Act of 1973. The Rehabilitation Act of 1973 prohibits discrimination based on disability in all private and government entities receiving federal funds. Section 504 of the Rehabilitation Act of 1973 is the basis for much of the ADA; however, the ADA is far more expansive than Section 504 because public and private entities, regardless of whether they receive federal funding, cannot discriminate on the basis of a disability. The ADA does far more than traditional civil rights legislation because it not only defines persons with disabilities as a protected class but also requires reasonable accommodations for people with disabilities. Reasonable accommodations are adjustments made that help a person with a disability do a job, attend school, or conduct some other related activity. No other protected class of people receives this kind of treatment under civil rights law (Pardeck, 1998).

The ADA has brought about attitudinal and behavioral changes toward persons with disabilities. These changes have helped to integrate people with disabilities into society. Shapiro (1993) concludes that persons with disabilities no longer want to simply receive subsides from the government; as able persons do, they wish to work. Research clearly concludes that the employment rate among persons with disabilities has been persistently low for the past several decades; a major goal of the ADA is to stop job discrimination against persons with disabilities (Pardeck, 1998).

The intent of this chapter is to discuss the impact of the ADA on family health in social work policy and practice. The chapter stresses that the ADA is a complicated law and that social workers must be aware of these complexities to ensure that they do not violate the rights of persons with disabilities. The ADA has helped to empower persons with disabilities; this empowerment has resulted in numerous changes that have improved the lives of people with disabilities.

## *DISCRIMINATION AND DISABILITY*

Congressional research leading to the passage of the ADA found that persons with disabilities are discriminated against in virtually every aspect of American life. Congressional findings reported that persons with disabilities had high rates of unemployment and poverty, low graduation rates from high school and college, and high levels of dependency on government programs (Pardeck, 1998). Research and testimonies presented to Congress noted that persons with disabilities are one of the most discriminated against groups in the United States (Pardeck, 1998).

For a person to be defined as disabled under the ADA, he or she must meet one or more of the following tests or prongs (ADA, 1990, p. 6). The person must

1. have a physical or mental impairment that substantially limits one or more of the major life activities, or
2. have a record of such an impairment, or
3. be regarded as having such an impairment.

Major life activities include but are not limited to walking, speaking, seeing, hearing, breathing, learning, working, reproduction, and caring for oneself (Pardeck, 1998).

The ADA does not provide a list of specific disabilities; the reason for not providing such a list was noted in a 1989 report (ADA, 1989, p. 22) from the United States Senate:

> It is not possible to include in the (ADA) legislation a list of all the specific conditions, diseases, or infections that would constitute physical or mental impairments because of the difficulty of ensuring the comprehensiveness of such a list, particularly in light of the fact that new disorders may develop in the future. The term includes, however, such conditions, diseases and infections as orthopedic, visual, speech, and hearing impairment, cerebral palsy, epilepsy, muscular dystrophy, multiple sclerosis, infections with the human immunodeficiency virus (HIV), cancer, heart disease, diabetes, mental retardation, emotional illness, and specific learning disabilities.

The definition of a disability under the ADA is aimed at changing the traditional stereotypes about persons with disabilities (Pardeck, 1998). Under the ADA, the term *disability* defines obvious impairments but also includes persons with a record of an impairment or being regarded as having an impairment. The second and third parts of the definition of a disability involve extremely complex legal issues, which means training and education are critical for agency employees to understand their obligations under the ADA (Pardeck, 1998). Social workers and other human service workers must realize that discrimination based on a record of an impairment or regarding someone as having an impairment when he or she does not is discriminatory behavior under the ADA.

## *HARRIS PUBLIC OPINION POLL AND THE ADA*

According to a recent Harris poll (1999), Americans overwhelmingly support civil rights for persons with disabilities. The 1999 Harris poll found the following:

1. Ninety percent of Americans who are aware of the ADA support and approve of it.
2. Two-thirds of all Americans have read or heard about the ADA.
3. Seventy-five percent of all Americans think that the benefits to people with disabilities are worth the additional costs to businesses and government.
4. More than eighty percent of Americans feel that creating opportunities for those with disabilities will decrease welfare roles and increase employment opportunities.
5. Ninety-four percent of Americans believe employers should not discriminate against any qualified candidate with a disability.
6. Eighty-five percent of Americans agree that employers with more than fifteen workers should make reasonable accommodations for employees with disabilities.
7. Ninety-one percent of Americans want to see public transportation made more accessible to disabled people.
8. Ninety-five percent of Americans agree that public places such as hotels, restaurants, theaters, stores, and museums must not discriminate against visitors with disabilities.
9. Eighty-six percent of Americans feel that government must offer home care services that allow more people with disabilities to live at home instead of in nursing homes.

## CASE STUDY: MARY ANN AND THE AMERICANS WITH DISABILITIES ACT

The following offers a case focusing on Mary Ann, a social worker, who was discriminated against in an employment situation based on her history of a disability, cancer. As noted earlier, the ADA defines a person with a disability as someone who has a physical or mental impairment that substantially limits one or more major life activities, who has a record of an impairment, or who is regarded as having an impairment. Mary Ann was employed by a large for-profit social work agency.

### Cancer and Employment Discrimination

For many cancer survivors, job discrimination is often worse than fighting the disease. It is estimated that 25 percent of survivors of cancer experience some form of job discrimination (Pardeck, 1994).

Cancer survivors often experience job discrimination because of stereotypes and myths. One common belief about cancer survivors is that they have high rates of absenteeism in the workplace due to long-term medical problems; no basis for this belief exists. Many employers have a traditional view of cancer; they simply think cancer must result in death. Employers often do not realize that many cancers can be cured or controlled. If given a chance, cancer survivors can be productive employees. More than 8 million cancer survivors live in the United States; survivors thus represent a large minority group that has historically experienced job discrimination (Pardeck, 1996).

### The Organizational Setting and a Discrimination Case

Mary Ann, as noted, worked in a large for-profit social work agency. Similar to many large social work organizations, the agency was highly bureaucratic and generally had a long history of lacking sensitivity to diversity and civil rights. Cases of discrimination in the agency were reported not only on the basis of disability but also regarding race and gender. The agency in one case spent more than $150,000 defending a charge of ethnic discrimination, and lost. Other cases of discrimination were settled discreetly and out of view of the public. Employees in the agency described the administrative hierarchy as being stuck in a dated mentality toward civil rights. The agency had little tolerance for dissent, and the internal due process mechanism for employees was less than effective.

A number of administrators achieved their rank in the agency on the basis of nepotism. Given this fact, many of the administrators were less than competent and had a vested interest in protecting each other's positions, even if civil rights laws were knowingly violated.

The previously mentioned discrimination case in the agency based on ethnicity provides insight into how the organization reacted when challenged in the area of employment discrimination. The case became public knowledge through the local media. The coverage of the case in the newspaper made it obvious that the administrators in the agency would protect one another at almost any cost. It was also clear that the agency had little understanding of civil rights laws or employment rights in general. Even after settling the case with the employee, the agency made few changes in its employment procedures (Pardeck, 1996).

The social worker in the case, Mary Ann, had obtained a master's of social work degree. Mary Ann, as noted earlier, had a history of cancer and was denied a supervisory position because of this history. A number of key administrators were well aware of Mary Ann's history of cancer. One high-ranking administrator who happened to not be aware of her history of cancer asked if she would be interested in the promotion even before it was advertised publicly. Mary Ann told the administrator she would be interested; however, she stated to the administrator that she had left a prior position of similar rank in another social work agency because of complications related to the cancer recovery process. Mary Ann felt that once the administrator learned of her history of cancer, this official was no longer interested in promoting her to the supervisory position. In fact, a fellow social worker who was a member of the committee that hired Mary Ann was asked by the administrator if he knew she had a history of cancer before the organization hired her (Pardeck, 1996).

The initial strategy used by Mary Ann was to work within the organizational structure by discussing the discrimination she felt she was experiencing with the equal employment officer (EEO). The goal of meeting with the EEO was to see if the problem could be corrected related to her application for the supervisory position. Another goal was to explore ways that the agency might be more sensitive to issues related to disabilities and to ensure that the ADA was being implemented appropriately. After a discussion with the EEO, Mary Ann concluded that the agency was not willing to correct its discriminatory acts against her. It also became clear to her that using the internal due process mechanism would prove fruitless.

Mary Ann had always received the highest job performance rankings possible within the agency. However, when Mary Ann officially applied for the supervisory position, she was not even granted an interview. A key informant involved in the promotion process concurred that Mary Ann's history of cancer probably played a role in her being denied the promotion. The key informant, however, did add that Mary Ann's references from her prior job were distorted by administrators within the agency. This distortion allowed those involved in the selection process to justify their actions of not promoting her to the position. Since Mary Ann's work record with the agency was excellent, she felt that the distortion of references from her prior job was the agency's strategy to justify its actions of nonpromotion. Mary Ann's work history prior to coming to the organization was also excellent.

Because many of the administrators in the agency were hired on the basis of nepotism and not merit, their reaction to Mary Ann's discussion with the EEO was negative and less than sophisticated. Historical information on prior challenges to the agency based on violations of civil rights law suggested that the agency would spend a great deal of time and resources defending itself even when obvious civil rights violations had occurred.

Mary Ann decided to file a discrimination complaint with the U.S. Equal Employment Opportunity Commission (EEOC) under the ADA. The complaint filed alleged that Mary Ann was a highly qualified candidate for the supervisory position. Not only was she not appointed to the position, the agency even denied her an interview. Mary Ann argued that the agency's discriminatory actions were because she had a history of cancer (Pardeck, 1996).

The EEOC's investigation, which took nearly one year, concluded that discrimination had occurred in Mary Ann's case. The EEOC claimed the organization's stated nondiscriminatory reason for not granting an interview, a weak reference, was a pretext for discrimination based on disability.

## ASSESSMENT IMPRESSIONS

The following are defenses used against a charge of employment discrimination under the ADA. A brief assessment of each of these helps one to understand how Mary Ann's discrimination complaint was found to have merit (Pardeck, 1998).

### Defenses

The ADA identifies five basic defenses used by employers to defend a discrimination employment complaint based on disability:

1. *Disparate treatment:* Disparate treatment means treating an individual differently on the basis of his or her disability. A defense to such a charge is that the actions taken by the employer were based on legitimate, nondiscriminatory reasons that are not pretextual, such as unsatisfactory job performance.
2. *Disparate impact selection:* In this context, disparate impact means that selection criteria, although uniformly applied, have an adverse impact on a person with a disability. Such criteria are permissible only when job related and consistent with business necessity and no reasonable accommodation is available. Where selection criteria include a safety requirement that an individual not pose a direct threat in the workplace, the employer must illustrate that this requirement is job related and consistent with business necessity.
3. *Disparate impact, nonselection:* This kind of disparate impact means that nonselection criteria such as employer policies, although uniformly applied, have an adverse impact on persons with disabilities. Such criteria are permissible only when job related and consistent with business necessity.
4. *Undue hardship:* Undue hardship may be raised, for example, as a defense to a charge that an employer failed to provide a reasonable accommodation for an employee.
5. *Conflict with other federal laws:* Where other federal laws may require or prohibit an action in conflict with the ADA requirements, the employer's efforts to comply with these conflicts can be a defense.

The EEOC and the court system generally use the same legal proofs as those employed under Title VII for discrimination cases based on race and other protected classes. The case law that has developed around legal rules related to the Rehabilitation Act of 1973 have also been the source for EEOC court decisions related to the ADA.

The proof scheme resulting from the *McDonnell Douglas v. Green* case is typically utilized for ADA employment discrimination cases (Greenlaw and Kohl, 1996). Following is a discussion of this case.

Green was laid off from his job as a result of his employer reducing its workforce. Green was a longtime civil rights activist, and he subsequently charged that he was laid off because he was an African American and an activist.

Green, in his protest against his former employer McDonnell Douglas, attempted to block the plant's five main access roads during rush hour in an attempt to prevent employees from entering. Green was arrested and fined for his actions.

A few weeks after Green's protest and his arrest, McDonnell Douglas advertised for "qualified mechanics"; Green applied. Green's application was rejected for his participation in the protest. He filed a charge of discrimination with the EEOC, charging the company would not hire him because he was an African American.

Green's case was appealed to the U.S. Supreme Court. As result of his appeal to the Supreme Court, a schema of both the proper order and nature of proofs in civil rights cases resulted. First, a plaintiff must present a prima facie case. Establishing a prima facie case entails four steps.

1. The plaintiff must show that he or she falls within a protected class. Green was black and thus was protected by race.
2. The plaintiff must show he or she was qualified for a position.
3. The individual must be rejected for the position.
4. The plaintiff must show that he or she was rejected for the job and the employer continued to seek applicants with similar qualifications to the plaintiff's.

If the prima facie case is established, the employer must show a legitimate nondiscriminatory reason for the employee's rejection. The plaintiff must then be given the opportunity to show the employer's nondiscriminatory reason was in fact a pretext for discrimination (Greenlaw and Kohl, 1996).

Mary Ann filed a discrimination complaint based on disparate treatment. Her complaint with the EEOC charged that she was treated differently from other applicants because of her disability. Using the *McDonnell Douglas v. Green* legal proofs, she was able to establish a prima facie case and ultimately proved that the distorted reference from her former employer was used as a pretext for discrimination based on disability, a history of cancer.

## *PROBLEM SOURCES AND MANIFESTATIONS*

Supervisors and employees in social work agencies must realize a number of traditional employment practices are no longer legal under the ADA. For example, it was a common practice in the past to ask a job applicant about his or her medical history; this is no longer legal. The following list covers activities social work employers in for-profit agencies cannot do (U.S. Equal Employment Opportunity Commission and U.S. Department of Justice, 1991, Section vii, pp. 2-3).

1. An application form cannot make inquiry regarding whether the person has a disability, ask how an individual became disabled or the prognosis of the disability, or how often the individual will need treatment or leave as a result of a disability. The employer may, however, state the attendance requirements for a position and ask the applicant if this requirement can be met.
2. A qualified person with a disability cannot be disqualified for a position because of the individual's inability to perform nonessential or marginal functions of a position.
3. Employment decisions must be based on facts applicable to individual applicants or employees and not on the basis of presumptions as to what a class of individuals with disabilities can or cannot do.
4. An individual with a disability cannot be assigned limited job duties based on a presumption of what is best for the individual or about the ability of the individual to perform certain tasks.

5. Employment of an applicant cannot be denied based on generalized fears about the safety of the applicant or higher rates of absenteeism.
6. A qualified individual with a disability must have equal access to health and life insurance and may not be subject to different terms of insurance based on the disability alone, if the disability does not impose increased risks.
7. Employment tests given to eligible applicants or employees who have sensory, manual, or speaking impairments must be adjusted to allow the applicant or employee to illustrate his or her skills.
8. Employers cannot use standards, criteria, or methods of administration that are not job related and consistent with business necessity and have the effect of discriminating or perpetuating discrimination.
9. Employers cannot restrict the employment opportunities, or segregate into separate work areas or into separate lines of advancement, qualified individuals with disabilities based on stereotypes and myths about disabilities.
10. An employer cannot deny an employment opportunity to an individual with a disability because of a slightly increased risk to the health or safety of others. The risk can be considered only when it poses a significant risk to others. Speculation is not sufficient.

## *INTERVENTION SKILLS*

The ADA is grounded in a human rights perspective. It is aimed at an oppressed group, persons with disabilities, who have been denied equal opportunity to participate in American society.

Under the ADA, persons with disabilities are viewed as a minority group. This perspective suggests that if a person with a disability is poor, it is less a result of a personal inadequacy than of a discriminatory society. Consequently, the adjustment to a disability is not merely a personal trouble but one that requires the larger community to change its views concerning persons with disabilities; the community must also remove the obstacles it has placed in the way of self-fulfillment for people with disabilities, including inaccessible transportation and architectural systems designed only for able persons (Karger and Stoesz, 1990).

Similar to other minority groups, people with disabilities have suffered tremendous discrimination (Ianacone, 1977). This discrimination is sometimes in the form of prejudice or patronizing attitudes; at other times it is the result of indifference. Regardless of the origin, the outcomes are the same: exclusion, segregation, and denial of equal treatment. The mandate of the ADA is correcting the numerous problems associated with discrimination against people with disabilities. Social workers grounded in a family health perspective will find advocacy an effective means for ensuring the ADA is implemented appropriately.

### *Advocacy and ADA*

Advocacy is a strategy for achieving social justice and empowering people. Advocacy helps individuals correct situations that are unjust. Social justice through advocacy requires the active participation of citizens who are vulnerable or disenfranchised; the family health practitioner plays a critical role in this process. Advocacy allows practitioners to achieve social justice through empowerment and responsible participation in the public realm (Lewis, 1992). A goal of the family health advocate is to speak on behalf of clients and to empower clients to speak on their own behalf in situations where their rights have been denied. Advocacy is a critical strategy for those who are grounded in a social justice approach to family health practice because it expands opportunities by protecting the interest of clients. Advocacy is a traditional role aimed at changing oppressing social environments, including systems that prevent individual growth and development (Pardeck, 1996).

McGowan (1987) suggests that advocacy can be conducted at two levels, *case advocacy* and *cause advocacy*. Case advocacy focuses on individuals. It involves the partisan intervention on behalf of a client or identified client group with one or more secondary institutions to secure or enhance needed services and resources (McGowan, 1987). Cause advocacy seeks to redress collective issues through social change efforts that include improving and implementing social policies.

## EVALUATION

The case of Mary Ann is an excellent example of a social worker using case advocacy on her own behalf. Given the fact that the ADA is aimed at preventing discrimination against persons with disabilities, this chapter has attempted to illustrate how the family health practitioner can use the ADA as an effective tool in the area of advocacy.

## REFERENCES

*Americans with Disabilities Act of 1989 (The)* (ADA) (1989). Washington, DC: Government Printing Office.
*Americans with Disabilities Act of 1990 (The)* (ADA) (1990). P. L. 101-336, 105 Stat. 327, 42 U.S.C., 12101 et seq.
Greenlaw, P. S. and Kohl, J. P. (1996). Proving ADA discrimination: The court's view. *Labor Law Journal, 46,* 376-383.
Harris, L., et al. (1999). *NOD/Harris survey of Americans with disabilities.* Washington, DC: National Organization on Disabilities.
Ianacone, B. P. (1977). Historical overview: From charity to rights. *Temple Law Quarterly, 50,* 953-960.
Karger, H. and Stoesz, D. (1990). *American social welfare policy.* New York: Longman.
Lewis, E. (1992). Social change and citizen action: A philosophical exploration for modern social group work. *Social Work with Groups, 14*(2), 23-34.
McGowan, B. G. (1987). Advocacy. In A. Minahan (Ed.), *Encyclopedia of social work,* Eighteenth edition, Volume 1 (pp. 89-95). Silver Spring, MD: National Association of Social Workers.
Pardeck, J. T. (1994). What you need to know about the Americans with Disabilities Act. *Coping,* July/August, 16-17.
Pardeck, J. T. (1996). *Social work practice: An ecological approach.* Westport, CT: Auburn House.
Pardeck, J. T. (1998). *Social work after the Americans with Disabilities Act: New challenges and opportunities for social service professionals.* Westport, CT: Auburn.
Shapiro, J. P. (1993). *No pity: People with disabilities forging a new civil rights movement.* New York: Times Book.
U.S. Equal Employment Opportunity Commission and U.S. Department of Justice. (1991). *Americans with Disabilities Act handbook.* Washington, DC: Government Printing Office.

Chapter 13

# Family Policy and Family Health

John T. Pardeck

The family system in the United States is under pressure. This pressure is reflected by an increasing number of families experiencing breakdown, an inadequate day care system for many parents, an economy that prevents a large percentage of families from meeting their basic needs, and a health and human services delivery system that fails millions of families. Clearly these conditions do not enhance family health as defined by this book. Complicating the many problems facing families is the reluctance of the national government to provide comprehensive family programs.

## *PROBLEM SOURCES AND MANIFESTATIONS*

Chung and Pardeck (1997) have identified a number of issues that help explain the lack of comprehensive programs within the United States. These include the following:

1. In the United States the individual is emphasized over the family system.
2. A preference for minimal government intervention in family life is a tradition within the United States.
3. The United States is a highly pluralistic society which has an extremely diverse value and belief systems. This diversity means it is very difficult to develop comprehensive social programs aimed at helping individual and families.

The first issue preventing the development of family policy and programs is grounded in the tradition of viewing the person as the focus of policy development. This view fits the needs of postindustrial American society. It also enhances the demands placed on individuals by a market economy. Capitalism is based on competition among individuals, not family systems. Furthermore, the market economy within the United States has not found a profit motive in supporting family systems. In others words, employers hire individuals, not families. Individualism is the basis for the political and economic systems in the United States; the tradition of placing the individual over the family system means the development of comprehensive family programs is extremely difficult both politically and economically.

The focus on individualism shapes the definition and cause of social problems. Most social programs in the United States attempt to solve social problems by treating individuals and exclude the important factors that enhance family health: the physical, mental, emotional, social, economic, cultural, and spiritual dimensions of family life. As long as programs treat only individuals and not the factors critical to family health, families will continue to be under pressure.

The second area preventing the development of family policy, the preference for minimal government intervention into family life, is related to the individualistic bias found in American society. The general view held by most persons is that the home and family are bastions of privacy. It is also assumed that government intervention is counterproductive to family life. The question of how government might be of service to the family is seldom raised (Pardeck, 2001).

Rice (1977) suggests that the reluctance to intervene into family life is partially grounded in the United States Constitution. Since the Constitution is completely silent on the subject of the family, Rice concludes that this omission was due to the founders' desire to avoid inherited social status as found in Europe. Consequently, the implicit contract is between the individual and the government, without reference to the family system. The Constitution's silence concerning the family has created a vacuum at the national level in terms of support for American families.

The final factor inhibiting the development of a family policy, pluralism, includes the diverse beliefs, values, norms, and attitudes found in American society. Pluralism tends to thwart efforts to achieve a consensus on what programs should be created to treat social problems.

For example, the American people overwhelmingly support the need for a national health insurance program; however, citizens have not been able to achieve a consensus through the political process defining what the program should consist of and what level of government should implement the program (Chung and Pardeck, 1997). Even though a national consensus on the need for national health insurance program exists, the pluralistic nature of American society has prevented agreement on how a universal health care program would be implemented and who would administer it.

Pluralism also results in incremental development of policy. Incrementalism slows the policymaking process, involves compromise for consensus building, and often results in modest modifications to existing programs. Lindblom (1959) concludes that comprehensive policy development is difficult not necessarily because of pluralism, but because of the limitations of the policymakers themselves. Lindblom argues that the technologies upon which social planning are based lack social scientific merit and offer little for developing rational policies not only at the national level but also at the state and local levels of government. However, one must note that many Western societies have been able to develop efficient comprehensive programs for families that include health care and social services; these programs suggest that Lindblom's analysis may be indicative of the U.S. policy development process but not necessarily of those found in other Western societies.

## *FAMILY POLICY SUPPORTING AMERICAN FAMILIES*

Most advocates of a national family policy in the United States believe that the components of such a policy should include a national health insurance program, a comprehensive income assistance program, and social services (Pardeck, 2001). The reality of the U.S. policymaking process suggests that family policy must evolve from existing policies and programs; these existing programs include those that offer health care to selected populations as well as income supports and social services.

History suggests that an interest in national health insurance in the United States has existed for some time. For example, in 1912, the Progressive Party under Theodore Roosevelt called for such a program in its national platform. The original Social Security Act of 1935 initially included national health insurance, but it was removed to ensure passage of the Act (Jansson, 2001). Since 1939, every Congress has introduced a national health insurance program. In 1949, President Truman urged the Congress to enact a comprehensive health insurance system in his State of the Union message. The most recent serious effort to introduce a national health insurance program was during Clinton's presidency. The United States continues to be one of the few industrialized nations that does not have national health insurance. National health insurance could be possible in the United States by building on existing medical programs. Two current programs, Medicare and Medicaid, have the potential to serve as the foundation for national health insurance; however, the financing and operation of these two programs are entirely different. Medicare is basically a program for retired persons over the age of sixty-five, and is financed through a premium paid by the insured and through the Social Security Act under Title 18. Medicaid is for the needy and those with low incomes, and is financed through federal and state governments as part of the Social Security Act under Title 19. Medicare and Medicaid might serve as the foundation for a comprehensive national health insurance program for all families. Both programs are national in scope and currently cover a large number of selected populations. Rather than creating an entirely new program, Medicare and Medicaid should be revised to open health coverage to all workers and their families not able to acquire health insurance from other sources.

Family income support programs are a necessity in postindustrial society. Advocates for family policy argue that income supports are particularly essential for families in need (Pardeck, 2001). At present, the United States is the only developed nation that does not have a coordinated economic support program for the family (Chung and Pardeck, 1997). The most recent effort aimed at creating such a program was in 1970s under then-President Nixon. Nixon during his presidency encouraged Congress to enact his Family Assistance Plan (FAP). FAP passed the House of Representatives but failed in the Senate. FAP was the last major effort at the national level aimed at creating comprehensive income supports for needy families. A form of national income supports affecting selected families currently exists in the Supplemental Security Income (SSI) program. SSI is designed for people in certain categories including the aged, and adults and children with disabilities. The SSI program ensures a minimum income level for these selected groups. SSI affects mainly low-income families by providing income support to family members who qualify for the program. SSI might serve as the foundation for a universal income support for all families in need. Since SSI is already national in scope, the major policy change would be to open the program to all needy families, thus ensuring that no family falls below a minimum income level.

The final component of a national family policy, comprehensive social services, must consider the unique political characteristics of American society. Since a national social services program designed for all families would be difficult to regulate and coordinate, an innovative approach might be the implementation of a voucher system. A voucher system would help to ensure that the current decentralized system becomes more accessible to families in need. A voucher/market system would allow families seeking social services to chose their own vendors. The vendors would be compensated by the appropriate government agency based on families using their services through vouchers. Requiring vendors to meet prescribed government regulations before compensation through vouchers would help to guarantee the quality of the services.

How realistic is a voucher delivery system? An example of a very large government voucher program is the GI Bill used by veterans from World War II up to the Vietnam War. Under the GI Bill, millions of veterans were granted the right to choose a college or vocational-training institution and the government provided funding for attendance. Food stamps and Medicaid are a current examples of voucher systems used by needy families and individuals. The basis for a national comprehensive family social services program now exists in the countless programs currently delivering social services to American families who qualify for these programs or who can afford their costs. By rechanneling the funding of these programs into a voucher system, a comprehensive social services program for the all families might be realized. A voucher system has the potential to effectively deliver services to families because it uses the existing programs and social service delivery system.

## *EVALUATION*

The factors preventing the movement toward a national family policy include

1. an emphasis on the individual over the family system,
2. a preference for minimal government intervention, and
3. pluralism.

These factors help to ensure that the policymaking process in the United States occurs incrementally. This process results in policymakers building on existing policies and programs when attempting to solve social problems (Pardeck, 1990).

The United States is one of the few developed nations that does not have a national comprehensive health insurance and income support program for families. The programs that currently provide assistance to the family do so indirectly, and a national family policy has not been formed. Several existing programs have been suggested in this chapter as foundations for a comprehensive family policy that would include a national health insurance program, an income assistance program, and social services for families. Medicare and Medicaid are two programs that could serve as the foundation for national health insurance. The Supplemental Security Income program (SSI) provides income support for selected groups; this program has the potential to be modified into a comprehensive family income support program. It was proposed that the funding for the diverse and often overlapping social services be redirected into a comprehensive social services program for the family. The program would be based on a voucher system. Finally, family policy in the United States is underdeveloped if not nonexistent. The lack of family policy within the United States prevents many families from achieving optimal family health. This means the physical, mental, emotional, social, economic, cultural, and spiritual dimensions of family life continue to suffer.

## REFERENCES

Chung, W. S. and Pardeck, J. T. (1997). Explorations in a proposed national family policy for children and families. *Adolescence,* 32, 429-436.

Jansson, Bruce A. (2001). *The reluctant welfare state—American social welfare policies: Past, present, and future,* Fourth edition. Pacific Grove, CA: Brooks Cole.

Lindblom, C. E. (1959). The science of "muddling through." *Public Administration Review, 19,* 79-88.

Pardeck, J. T. (1990). An analysis of the deep social structure preventing the development of a national policy for children and families in the United States. *Early Child Development and Care, 57,* 23-30.

Pardeck, J. T. (2001). *Children's rights: Policy and practice.* Binghamton, NY: The Haworth Press.

Rice, M. (1977). *American family policy: Content and context.* New York: Family Service Association of America.

# SECTION III: REFLECTION, SUMMARY, AND CONCLUSION

Chapter 14

# The Utilities of the Family Health Approach When Working in a Family Education and Support Program

Katie Ellsworth

## *PROGRAM OVERVIEW*

Contrary to many chapters of this text, this chapter does not include a case study but rather a description of a program that utilizes the family health perspective. Of note, the program was originally developed from a more generic social work perspective but has unintentionally taken on the family health perspective. The Family Education and Support Program is a social service provided to any interested families currently living in this primarily midsized Midwestern city. The purpose of the program is to improve the development of all children in the county through the education of their parents. The focus is on the child's (or children's) intellectual, social, language, and motor development. Services range from support and encouragement to dramatic economic makeovers. Program components can be delivered from any level of practice and include such activities as home visits, group therapy, developmental screenings, and linkage to community resources. Services begin during the mother's pregnancy and can continue until the child enters kindergarten at age five. Put simply, this program does whatever it takes to further the development of these children and provide them with opportunities to succeed. Although the program has many set activities prepackaged for delivery to families, parent educators also provide services that are tailored to fit the individual needs of each family system. It is a voluntary program, provided at no cost to all interested families. Consequently, a diversity of clientele exists across many demographic variables (e.g., socioeconomic status, family type, age, race, and level of need).

## FAMILY HEALTH PERSPECTIVE

The family health perspective is an innovative melding of social work and social science knowledge into a more comprehensive and therefore more beneficial assessment and intervention package than previously conceptualized in the social work literature. A multitude of empirical support from a number of disciplines is found for such a conceptualization (Bomar, 1996; Campbell, 1986; Carter and McGoldrick, 1989; Danielson, Hamel-Bissell, and Winstead-Fry, 1993; Edelman and Mandle, 1998; McDaniel, Hepworth, and Doherty, 1992; McNight, 1997; Pardeck and Yuen, 1999; Pardeck et al., 1998; Pender, 1996; Thompson and Pardeck, 2000). Family health "is a state of holistic well-being of the family system. It is manifested by the developmental of, and continuous interaction among, the physical, mental, emotional, social, cultural, and spiritual dimensions of the family, which results in the holistic well-being of family members" (School of Social Work, Southwest Missouri State University, 1996, p. 1). It is a comprehensive and inclusive perspective that is, in many cases, unwittingly utilized by most social workers in practice today. The approach has many benefits.

## COMPARISON OF THE FAMILY HEALTH PERSPECTIVE AND THE FAMILY EDUCATION AND SUPPORT PROGRAM

### *Philosophical Similarities*

Although the assessment and intervention approaches of the Family Education and Support Program were developed based on the generalist perspective, the needs and the philosophies of the perspective and program are very similar. Clearly, parenting and children's issues can have a tremendous impact on the family system. Considering each dimension of the family health approach can help make intervention most effective. For example, families may experience strain because of child-rearing issues such as child care, preschool, and health care costs. The family may rely on *spirituality* as a way of dealing with the responsibilities of caregiving. *Physically,* the families may experience fatigue and exhaustion in their attempts to meet the needs of their children and routine outside demands such as employment and the extended family. The variety of *emotional* reactions of families to parenthood and children's development includes excitement, frustration, anxiety, confusion, desperation, and others. *Socially,* they may have little contact with others because of a lack of knowledge about activities, time constraints, or family pressures. *Mentally,* the responsibilities of being a parent can result in anxiety and in some cases depression. Finally, a family's *cultural* background can be a great influence on the beliefs, attitudes, and practices related to raising children.

Attempting to understand and assist families and their members requires a comprehensive assessment and intervention package. The Family Education and Support Program uses a family health perspective as it highlights the importance of the family in the developmental process.

## Similarities of Services

According to Pardeck and colleagues (1998), nine intervention skills used by family health practitioners are:

1. Developmental assessment
2. Resource linkage
3. Supportive intervention
4. Confrontive intervention
5. Empowering framework
6. Using social learning approaches
7. Recognizing the level of prevention and readiness for change
8. Utilization of the family unit as a change agent
9. Understanding and assessing the construction of the client's reality (social constructionist approach).

The Family Education and Support Program social workers utilize all of these skills in their practice.

The nature of this education and support program with young families quite obviously lends itself to a physical and mental *developmental assessment* of the child. Of course, what is also necessary is a developmental work-up of the family. For example, Carter and Mc-Goldrick (1989) and others have created descriptions of family life cycles and developmental stages throughout the life of the family. For example, when families add new members, adjustments must be made to the marital system, the sharing of daily tasks, including child rearing, and a realignment of relationships. Both the child's and family's assessments must be placed in the context of the social, economic, spiritual, and other environments in which the family finds itself.

*Resource linkage* is an important component of this program, as families often do not have the knowledge of community resources available to them. An assessment can be done with each family to include each individual, the family system, and the social network in an effort to focus services and information on parent interests and needs. Parent educators pay special attention to the role that larger ecosystems play in family functioning when incorporating the family health model. Families are affected by countless outside sources such as parental employment, child care, extended family, neighbors, schools, and religious organizations. Families are also involved in programs and agencies such as Medicaid, Women, Infants, and Children (WIC), division of family services, probation, and parole. These larger ecosystems and their relationship to each family help determine activities, beliefs, roles, attitudes, and behaviors within the family system. Having knowledge of this information is critical for the parent educator to provide the most beneficial services. Therefore, a key component of this program is collaboration with other professionals and organizations. This knowledge and linkage with other social work professionals and agencies *empowers* the family by mobilizing resources around the family's strengths. The parent educator works together with others to provide the most comprehensive services to meet families' needs. Collaboration with and referrals to health professionals, early childhood special education, division of family services, speech-language programs, schools, WIC, shelters, and emergency food and clothing agencies are common. Each professional utilizes his or her particular expertise with the family's best interest in focus.

*Supportive intervention* is also necessary; empathy and appreciation of the differences in families develops strong working relationships. To shape behaviors, educators regularly use *social learning approaches* such as modeling positive interaction with children and reading books during visits.

Of course, the professional needs to be honest in assessments, and honest *confrontation* of family members as the need arises promotes effective family health practice.

*Recognizing the readiness for change* is important for both the education and support program as well as the family health perspective. Unless family members are psychologically ready, willing, and interested in effecting a change, the intervention will not be successful. A parallel in medicine occurs when a physician prescribes a medication that could cure a patient, but the patient refuses to take the medicine. The patient will not recover and the physician is powerless to force the patient to comply. It is important, therefore, to have an intervention plan that is consistent with the client family's wishes. As motivation increases, so does the success rate.

Finally, to provide services based on each family's needs, it is critical for educators to utilize the family health approach by gaining the *family's perspective* of the situation. Each family member and the family as a collective has a unique interpretation of the problems and needs. Assessments and interventions based on traditional formulas or procedures are very unlikely to succeed unless the family interprets their needs as consistent with that perspective.

Throughout the entire process, successful intervention must remain focused on the family as the source of strength and the *change agent* for effective practice.

## *FAMILY HEALTH PRACTITIONER ROLES*

Pardeck (1996) and Pardeck and Yuen (1997) list six roles a family health social worker must adopt to be successful practitioners: conferee, enabler, broker, mediator, advocate, and guardian.

Using the family health approach, the social worker is "part of" the helping process. The parent educator also adheres to this perspective as she or he takes on the role of facilitator within the family. Instead of acting as an outsider, the educator works to build a relationship with the family system by listening, providing support and encouragement, and giving information. The educator is aware that a family's behavior, attitudes, and actions can be greatly affected by such interaction and modeling over time, as trust and rapport are established. This *enables* the educator to influence, structure, or otherwise change events and variables that enhance system functioning.

Family health intervention skills are also evident in the parent educator position within this program. An integral part of this program is its focus on family strengths and strategies to empower parents. The parent educator treats participants with respect, highlights strengths to increase confidence, and provides child development information so that parents can make informed decisions about their children. Therefore, the parent educator needs to be competent in multiple roles. As a *conferee,* the educator can provide support through problem-solving issues such as sibling conflict, the display of inappropriate behavior, and sleep difficulties. As a *broker,* the educator provides parents information and linkages to community resources that may be of assistance, such as a community child care resource agency, WIC, area emergency assistance organizations, Medicaid, and speech-language and developmental disability services. With so many people, resources, and other variables impacting the family, the educator as *mediator,* needs to reconcile opposing or disparate points of view. The goal is unitary action. In yet another role, an educator's *advocacy* efforts can be of great importance in working toward policy changes for funding on the legislative level. Advocacy on behalf of a client's interest or need is especially important where the client is reluctant or possesses inadequate resources. Finally, as *guardian,* the educator performs a social control function or even takes protective action when the competency of a client is inadequate. It is a role educators may play often with this client type (incompetents).

## *CONCLUSION*

The challenges and questions involved with parenting can be overwhelming at times, and having support and assistance through those periods can be of tremendous value. By working with the family system and emphasizing a holistic focus to services, family health care workers can ensure that families benefit from all the information, resources, and support the program offers. Workers attend to each family's circumstances with a service designed to fit the individual family's interests and needs.

## REFERENCES

Bomar, P. J. (1996). *Nurses and family health promotion: Concepts, assessment, and interventions,* Second edition. Philadelphia, PA: W.B. Saunders Company.

Campbell, T.L. (1986). Family's impact on health: A critical review and annotated bibliography. *Family systems medicine, 4,* 135-328.

Carter, B. and McGoldrick, M. (1989). *The changing family life cycle.* Boston, MA: Allyn & Bacon.

Danielson, C.B., Hamel-Bissell, B., and Winstead-Fry, P. (1993). *Families, health, and illness: Perspectives on coping and intervention.* St. Louis, MO: Mosby.

Edelman, C. L. and Mandle, C.L. (1998). *Health promotion throughout the lifespan,* Fourth edition. St. Louis, MO: Mosby.

McDaniel, S.H., Hepworth, J., and Doherty, W.J. (1992). *Medical family therapy: A biopsychosocial approach to families with health problems.* New York: Basic Books.

McNight, J.L. (1997). A 21st-century map for healthy communities and families. *Families in Society,* March/April, 117-127.

Pardeck, J.T. (1996). *Social work practice: An ecological approach.* Westport, CT: Auburn House.

Pardeck, J. T. and Yuen, F.K.O. (1997). A family health approach to social work practice. *Family Therapy, 24*(2), 115-128.

Pardeck, J. T. and Yuen, F.K.O. (1999). *Family health: A holistic approach to social work practice.* Westport, CT: Auburn House.

Pardeck, J.T., Yuen, F.K., Daley, J.G., and Hawkins, C.L. (1998). Social work assessment and intervention through family health practice. *Family Therapy, 25*(1), 25-39.

Pender, N.J. (1996). *Health promotion in nursing practice,* Third edition. Stamford, CT: Appleton and Lange.

School of Social Work, Southwest Missouri State University (1996). A working paper on family health. Springfield, MO: Author.

Thompson, R. and Pardeck, J. T. (2000). An exploration of the themes and content of family health in the social work literature. *Early Child Development and Care, 161,* 15-31.

Chapter 15

# The Biopsychosocial Model of Pain Management

Mark J. Kellen

## INTRODUCTION

Pain is a universal condition affecting all of humanity. The International Association for the Study of Pain (IASP, 1986) defines pain as "an unpleasant sensory and emotional experience associated with actual and potential tissue damage, or described in terms of such damage" (p. S217). As long as humans have recorded history, the horrors of headaches, abscessed teeth, cutaneous ulcerations, and tumors have been recounted. The twentieth century saw rapid medical advances in the diagnosis and treatment of painful conditions. The average individual can easily eliminate a headache with aspirin or acetaminophen. Tooth decay is prevented by proper brushing, flossing, and dental care. Bacterial infections are readily treated with a wide array of modern antibiotics. Tumors are painlessly resected using general or regional anesthesia in modern operating rooms. These and many other current medical treatments would have been looked on as magic only 200 years ago.

With this wonderful armamentarium of laboratory tests, X rays, nerve tests, muscle tests, and the like, we should be able to diagnose and treat any painful condition that exists. This is the biomedical model of pain management. All a physician needs to do is identify the problem, institute the appropriate treatment, and the patient is miraculously cured. This model does indeed work in the majority of cases.

It was recognized in the 1950s that a large number of patients unfortunately do not seem to have an identifiable problem, or a problem is identified but the usual treatments do not work. To address this, the first multidisciplinary pain clinics appeared in the 1960s. Engel developed the concept of the biopsychosocial model of medicine in 1977 and shortly thereafter applied it to pain management, thus emphasizing the importance of the whole person in the treatment plan for chronic pain conditions.

To understand how the mind functions, it is important to understand pain and suffering. Pain is a physical experience. Nerve endings are stimulated, and a signal is sent to the brain. Suffering is how we respond to the pain, and it is solely a function of our emotions. My grandmother broke her wrist but insisted on going to church before moving on to the hospital. Certainly pain existed, but no suffering, and my grandmother sat quietly.

On the other hand we have all seen people with minor cuts who will cry, scream, and tell everyone they meet how horrible they feel. A classic stereotype—that husbands complain and mope around the house with the mildest cold while wives go through labor and delivery of a child all the while performing all the work expected of them—further elucidates the importance suffering plays in the human experience. These examples demonstrate that a large part of our response to pain is emotional and within our control. Many other examples of suffering (also known as pain behaviors) occur, and we watch for these during patient interviews.

Thus, we turn to what is known as the biopsychosocial model of pain management. This represents a full circle back to the concept of physician as healer. Until the twentieth century, very few truly effective treatments existed. A physician was revered for the compassion toward and care of the sick person. The technological advances of the twentieth century led us down a new road. We slowly lost the concept of treating the human being and evolved into treating gallbladders, lungs, or hearts.

For confirmation of this concept we can look at popular films such as *The Doctor* (1991) with actor William Hurt, in which the doctor suddenly finds himself as "the laryngeal cancer" rather than "the person with laryngeal cancer." A more recent film concerning the same concept from a different perspective is *Patch Adams* (1999) with actor Robin Williams. As Lang et al. (1999) state, the proper emphasis in a pain management clinic must be biopsychosocial when dealing with chronic nonmalignant pain, using a biomedical model when it seems appropriate. They also point out that physicians who use the biopsychosocial model need to be recruited to pain management fellowships.

The most important part of using this model is teaching the patient independence. In the usual medical encounter, the patient is the passive recipient of care; this usually reinforces the patient's negative attitudes and behaviors. The biopsychosocial model works toward making the patient an active participant in the care plan. In my own practice, I also refer to the patient as the "boss," and to myself as an information source. An analogy with parenting (kindness, compassion, and yet firm guidance) is very applicable to managing patients with chronic nonmalignant pain. I never allow a patient to use the phrase, "What are you going to do for me?" Properly phrased, the question should be stated, "What can you help me do for myself?"

Patients who fail the usual treatments are not malingerers. The biopsychosocial model of pain management acknowledges that pain is a physical symptom that arises due to known causes such as broken bones, strained muscles, or torn ligaments. Suffering is a function of our interpretation of the physical signals that reach our brain. Our ability to accept and move forward from these physical symptoms is heavily dependent on our psychological state. Our psychological state is influenced by how our parents raised us. We tend to grow strong if we were fortunate enough to have strong stable parents. Or we grow weaker if we experienced episodes of abuse, parental substance disorders, poor relationships, divorce, and so forth. As adults we can have spouses, family, or friends who lead us into healthy lifestyle choices, or who sit around continually telling us how we cannot succeed, or who inadvertently foster dependence.

This first case is fictional, but it demonstrates how family interactions, plus a medical condition, can develop into a patient suffering from a chronic pain syndrome. The last four cases are real.

## *CASE #1*

The patient, Alicia, is a thirty-year-old female married for ten years, with children ages eight, six, and four. Her husband, David, works constantly, provides wonderful financial and emotional support for the children, but forgets about Alicia. This is not a conscious decision. Then one day, Alicia hurts her back while lifting and suddenly David sees need, so he steps in by doing all the work around the house and providing meals in bed and back rubs and massages. He is genuinely concerned for his wife, as he loves her very much, but he finds it difficult to discuss his feelings.

Alicia does less and less, and her pain grows and grows. She sees her primary physician, whose treatment fails; she then sees an orthopedic surgeon, who obtains an MRI (magnetic resonance imaging) showing a ruptured disc matching the pain symptoms. The orthopedic surgeon believes removing the disc will cure Alicia (the biomedical model). The surgery is scheduled, the disc is removed, and the pain is . . . still there.

Now the world changes, because the armor cracks and Alicia must be faking it. She is looked down upon by others who "beat their back problem." Her pain has persisted for a year now, and she has become dependent on multiple medications. Given her lack of activity, she has gained forty pounds. She is depressed and frustrated because her pain will not go away. Her husband is growing impatient. She feels unattractive. The children are complaining because she cannot do anything anymore. The downward spiral of pain, inactivity, and frustration leading to more pain is in full swing. Intimate relations between Alicia and David have not existed for months, and Alicia lands in the pain center crying over her "pain," sure that her husband is ready to leave.

Where do we begin when treating such a horrible condition? We begin by moving to the proper model of care in these situations: the biopsychosocial model. The first visit involves a thorough history and physical to be certain that previous care providers missed nothing serious. With most cases nothing serious is found, and the patient is referred for psychological support. In these sessions, all aspects of the patient's life both before and after the injury are examined and put into perspective, so the patient can see how each part of her life led up to her present situation and how these stresses cause suffering over and above the pain.

Once the patient can accept that suffering is something she can control, the physical aspects of her pain such as poor nutrition, inactivity, loss of the ability to sleep, and appropriate pain control can be addressed. Thus the patient is on her way to recovery, after the "condition" was poorly controlled for such a long time.

The first case is presented so that the subtle points are obvious. In the clinic setting patients do not wear signs advertising their personal problems. The clinician has to dig for them, and even then the patient may not share personal problems until communication over a number of visits establishes an element of trust. Some of the best medical exams are performed while talking to the patient about family, hobbies, interests, or the weather. In this way, the patient drops his or her guard and a true picture of the soul can emerge. Motions of the extremities are easily evaluated, as gesturing becomes relaxed and natural. The true degree of suffering becomes apparent, as the tears fade away with the distraction of conversation.

Family history should be covered both from a medical perspective and a social perspective, as social learning can play just as great a role in pain problems as genetics. Perceived disability is always high in relation to the physical findings; thus, determination of what has led the patient to develop such a low sense of self-control or self-esteem is essential. Finally, realistic goals that emphasize rehabilitation rather than cure must be established. It is often unrealistic for the patient to expect 100 percent pain relief; it is equally unrealistic for the physician to expect to cure everyone.

## *CASE #2*

Sarah is a fifty-five-year-old female with a thirteen-year history of intermittent back pain, controlled easily with traditional medical treatments. There were no complaints until two months prior to her first visit to the pain center, when her back began to ache after a few strenuous days working at her restaurant job. Her husband died a few years earlier, and she has had few interactions with the rest of her family since then. In addition, Sarah had been diagnosed with breast cancer a year ago and has just finished radiation and chemotherapy. She also has greatly diminished social interactions with friends and co-workers.

On examination, the patient had some muscles that were sore and the possibility existed of some problems with the nerves in her back, but the most significant aspect of her history and physical was that she frequently cried while we discussed her situation. We referred Sarah for counseling and at the same time commenced medical therapy aimed at her physical complaints. Over the course of two months Sarah complained of less and less pain and at the same time became more positive in her thoughts. She began to spend more time with the friends she had been avoiding. She started to understand how the difficulties in her life contributed to suffering (something we control), and all these ideas combined with appropriate medical therapy led to the resolution of her symptoms.

We had good success with this patient because the social factors involved in her complaints were readily apparent and appropriate counseling was instituted early. Jacobson et al. (1997) stated that chronic nonmalignant pain is conceptualized as the result of complex and inseparable interactions involving biological, psychological, social, and cultural factors. The focus shifts from pain as a biological process to the analysis of pain as experienced by the patient and communicated to others. Biomedical interventional techniques are considered to be of limited use because it is recognized that chronic pain is rarely caused by nerve activity alone. These statements are an appropriate summary of this patient's circumstances. Medications and injections were used, but had we failed to address her growing social isolation, her symptoms might not have been alleviated at all.

## *CASE #3*

Sharon is a fifty-three-year-old female with a twenty-year history of severe headaches and multiple muscular complaints. All known medial therapies had failed; crying during the initial interviews was common. Due to arguments with the staff, she had been discharged from another pain clinic and sent to us. We began injection therapy to facilitate medication withdrawal as well as to treat the possibility of a neuropathic process. This worked well but did not last longer than seven to ten days, prompting a more detailed psychosocial history.

It became apparent that the headaches correlated with family difficulties. An uncle had abused Sharon when she was younger, and she did not want to have anything to do with him. A brother kept insisting that she "bury the hatchet," thus creating more friction. Also, after a year of therapy, I learned that Sharon had reading and writing skills on a first-grade level. Our therapeutic goal was appropriate medications to control the headaches, combined with counseling to assist the patient in dealing with her family. Ultimately, medications should be tapered back as Sharon becomes mentally stronger. She has resisted attempts at counseling and improving her reading skills, and continues to use medication excessively.

This patient, after more than two years of interaction, continues to be a very difficult problem. She refused to seek counseling despite my best efforts to convince her of its importance, but did listen to my suggestions during our "medical follow-ups." She was also very slow to make the connection between family stress and her headache pattern. However, her case demonstrates that years of therapy, reassurance, and care continuity are neccesary for many such individuals. Jacobson and associates (1997) discusses patients exhibiting a complex array of features, characterized by depression, conflict with the medical legal systems, emotional issues, family dysfunction, and substance abuse problems. As a consequence, care-seeking is an integral aspect of the pain experience, and excessive health care use ensues. This patient exhibited all of this in her history.

Jacobson and associates (1997) also state that psychosocial factors predict health care use better than the number or severity of physical symptoms. Once again, the patient matches the description perfectly.

Roy (1986) has noted that deteriorating family relationships can be a tremendous stimulus for severe chronic headaches; thus we spent a great deal of time talking about family dynamics. I am optimistic that progress will eventually be made, as she is slowly involving herself in outside activities and standing up to difficult family members.

## CASE #4

Ruth is a thirty-three-year-old female with a two-year history of pelvic pain unresponsive to usual medical interventions up to and including surgery. On evaluation in the pain management center, we identified a muscular/ligamentous trigger point that completely relieved her pain with injection. Relief lasted approximately three weeks. We followed this procedure two more times with the same results. Upon calling for a fourth injection, Ruth exhibited enough trust to allow a rather detailed psychosocial history.

We uncovered multiple family difficulties (childhood), along with stress involving children and her work. Working together, patient and physician were able to alleviate a large percentage of the pain simply by educating Ruth about how she was focusing her life stress through physical complaints. These were apparently more socially acceptable for her than admitting she was emotionally distraught.

This case demonstrates the importance of listening, and Goodwin summarizes it best by stating: "When complete understanding is abandoned as a goal, the traditional tasks of the physician—listening, witnessing, and relieving suffering—will no longer be relegated to a small corner of medicine, the so-called art of medicine, but will be returned to the core of medical practice and medical education" (1997, p. 1400). As part of a pain management team, experts in counseling can assist the physician in helping patients such as this woman by aiding in the listening process. This case also demonstrates the assertion by Jacobson et al. (1997) that the primary role of the biopsychosocial anesthesiologist is physician-educator, not technical expert.

Unless judiciously delivered in an appropriate biopsychosocial context, nerve blocks are interventions that might help patients feel better in the short term, but which do not address the fundamental problem of being overwhelmed by the psychosocial consequences of chronic pain in the long term. It was very rewarding to hear this patient make the connection between her pain and her social situation by stating, after one of our counseling sessions, "I don't think I need the block anymore."

## CASE #5

Jim is a thirty-nine-year-old male with severe back spasm and pain who was resistant to counseling for the first few months but eventually agreed. He blamed his back problems on work, likely the source given his heavy-lifting requirements. However, through two different counselors it became apparent that Jim's childhood was exceedingly difficult. He grew up with an abusive alcoholic father and a passive unemotional mother. Jim eventually divorced his second wife seven months into our treatments. Every moment of his day was spent avoiding pain with short-term ideas. He ultimately left the clinic when we refused any further sedatives/controlled substances and injections.

This case serves as proof that not all patients can be helped, thus providing a sense of balance and realism to treatment expectations.

This particular patient demonstrated a number of classic problems with chronic nonmalignant pain. In addition, Jacobson and associates (1997) state that the risks of nerve block treatment are not confined to the physical complications of the procedure. Such treatment reinforces patient belief in biomedical procedure as a cure for any underlying abnormality. Further, biomedical treatment maintains expectations that the patient should be a passive recipient rather than an active participant in the process, and fosters the illusion that the primary problem in the patient's life is pain. I have rarely seen patients where this was better illustrated.

When the psychosocial factors, which are typically maintaining or exacerbating the patient's suffering, are neglected, the expensive, futile, and endless search for biomedical solutions is perpetuated (Jacobson et al., 1997). We once talked for forty-five minutes about why counseling and a healthy lifestyle would help him immensely, and that he needed to stop focusing on short-term quick fixes. Jim voiced understanding and then promptly asked, "Can I have a shot tomorrow?" This pattern had been repeating itself for a few weeks when he finally told us he did not want to see us anymore.

## CONCLUSION

This chapter provides an introduction to pain management as a medical discipline. It is fundamentally a multidisciplinary specialty in which physicians, counselors, physical therapists, nurses, chiropractors, and dietitians all work together toward the common goal of alleviating suffering in patients often felt to be beyond help by the traditional medical community.

Virtually any practitioner with skills related to human suffering can become a member of a pain management team. The practice is very difficult and requires individuals with patience, understanding, and superb listening skills; identifying and changing behaviors which have been ingrained for fifty years is challenging. However, it is also one of the most rewarding fields of practice, because the relief of suffering is by far the most important reason physicians began to practice thousands of years ago.

## REFERENCES

Engel, G. L. (1997). The need for a new medical model: A challenge to biomedicine. *Science, 196,* 129-136.

Goodwin, J. S. (1997). Chaos and the limits of biomedicine. *JAMA, 278,* 1399-1440.

International Association for the Study of Pain (IASP) (1986). Classification of chronic pain: Descriptions of chronic pain syndromes and definitions of pain terms. *Pain,* Suppl. 3, S217.

Jacobson, L., Mariano, A. J., Chabal, C., and Chaney, E. F. (1997). Beyond the needle: Expanding the role of anesthesiologists in the management of chronic nonmalignant pain. *Anesthesiology, 87,* 1210-1218.

Lang, S. A., Arraf, J., Tumber, P., and Shah, M. (1999). The role of the anesthesiologist in the management of chronic nonmalignant pain: A Canadian perspective. *Anesthesiology, 90,* 1237.

Roy, R. (1986). Marital conflicts and exacerbation of headache: Some clinical observations. *Headache, 26,* 360-364.

Chapter 16

# Family Health Social Work Practice: Summary, Problems, Focuses, Theories, and Intervention Skills

Francis K. O. Yuen
Gregory J. Skibinski

In 1997, Pardeck and Yuen discussed family health social work practice and explored the basic philosophical and theoretical underpinnings of that perspective. Pardeck and colleagues (1998) described the basics of the family health social work approach, including its guiding premises, models, and intervention skills. The book *Family Health: A Holistic Approach to Social Work Practice* (edited by Pardeck and Yuen, 1999) offers a wider discussion of the utilities of the family health social work approach. The following is a summary of some of the key concepts of the family health approach and its associated skills.

## *DEFINITION OF THE FAMILY*

A family is a system of two or more interacting persons who are either related by ties of marriage, birth, adoption, or who have chosen to commit themselves to each other as a unity for the common purpose of promoting the economic, physical, mental, emotional, social, cultural, and spiritual growth and development of the unit and each of its members (Pardeck and Yuen, 1997; Pardeck et al., 1998).

## DIMENSIONS OF THE FAMILY

Adapted and slightly modified from Pardeck and associates (1998, p. 28), the conceptualization of the family is developed upon the dimensions of nature, structure, and function.

### *Nature*

The nature of a family is its essential characteristics and qualities. The fundamental or primary unit of a society is the family. It is characterized by its unconditional concerns or commitments for the total well-being of its members and itself. People who come together and share these traits, characteristics, or qualities maximize the utilities of the family.

### *Structure*

Family structure is the invisible set of functional demands that organizes the ways in which family members interact. A family is a system that operates through transactional patterns. Repeated transactions establish patterns of how, when, and to whom to relate, and these patterns underpin the system. Transactional patterns influence family members' behaviors.

### *Function*

Family function comprises the activities necessary for realizing the family's common purpose, that is, promoting the economic, physical, mental, emotional, social, cultural, and spiritual growth and development of itself and each of its members. Thus, the functions of a family are intricately tied to the needs of the family as assessed by the family and the communities of which it is a member.

## DEFINITION OF HEALTH

Health is a state of holistic well-being. It means being connected in a fulfilling way with the natural and human world (Pardeck et al., 1998, p. 29).

## DEFINITION OF FAMILY HEALTH

Family health is a state of holistic well-being of the family system. Family health is manifested by the development of, and continuous interaction among, the economic, physical, mental, emotional, social, cultural, and spiritual dimensions of the family that results in its holistic well-being as well as that of its members.*

## FAMILY HEALTH INTERVENTION SKILLS

1. *Developmental assessment* (including individual, family, and social network) involves the use of biopsychosocial assessment with emphasis on the impact of health care settings on developmental concerns.
2. *Resource linkage* stresses finding and accessing resources with sensitivity to the political context of resource access and usage, the importance of formal and informal networking within the community, and the legal boundaries surrounding resource coordination.
3. *Supportive intervention* involves the effective use of empathy, building on relationship, and appreciating diversity.
4. *Confrontive intervention* entails recognizing when and how to confront within an empowerment framework.
5. *Empowering the client* is grounded in the strength perspective, an orientation inherent in family health social work practice that emphasizes multilevel interventions at the micro-, mezzo-, and macrolevels.
6. *Using social learning approaches* requires the application of techniques that are useful for shaping behaviors in individuals and families and enhancing cognitive restructuring.
7. *Recognizing the level of prevention and readiness for change* involves working at the primary, secondary, and tertiary levels of prevention and fitting interventions to the stage or readiness for change.

---

*This information is adapted and modified from School of Social Work, SMSU, 1996, p. 1. The information in the following section is adapted and modified from Pardeck and associates, 1998, p. 36.

8. *Utilization of the family unit as change agent* makes the family unit a force for change; an understanding of family communication, power dynamics, cohesion, and reality constructions is critical.
9. *Understanding and assessing the construction of a client's reality* requires basing assessment and intervention on a client's personal epistemology and perspective of a presenting problem.
10. *Advocating for the client* involves empowering clients in promoting change, taking social actions, and achieving social justice.

## *FAMILY HEALTH FOCUSES, THEORIES, AND SKILLS*

The family health approach is an integrated one that offers comprehensive intervention in family health social work practice. In this approach, the practitioners must become familiar with the conceptual and practical groundwork needed to work effectively with families. A rigorous process of family assessment, planning, implementation, and evaluation achieves goodness of fit between the family's assessed need and the family health social work interventions. Table 16.1 presents a display of intervention skills, practice theory, and problem focuses applicable to many areas of practice. This table is adapted from a document that the School of Social Work at Southwest Missouri State University (1998, pp. 3-8) submitted to the Council of Social Work Education as part of its response to an accreditation visit.

Basic family interviewing techniques include circular questioning, family-level probing, reframing, culture-sensitive questions, self-awareness in family interviews, negotiating, family structure clarifying, relationship building, contract development, process tracking, empowerment, time management, age-appropriate queries or activities, ethically bounded intervening, use of silence, and strategies for various "difficult" family behaviors.

Basic wellness techniques include recognizing level of prevention, readiness for change assessment, family resiliency building, family communication enhancement, blending individual and family wellness priorities, differentiating family issues from environmental issues, and advocating with systems external to family.

TABLE 16.1. Problem Focuses, Theoretical Foundations, and Practice Intervention Skills

| Problem Focuses and Opportunities | Practice Theories | Practice Intervention Skills |
|---|---|---|
| *PIE (Person-in-Environment) Clients Problem Complex*<br>Social functioning problems, type, severity, duration, and coping ability<br>Environmental problems, severity, and duration<br>Mental health problems<br>Physical health problems | Ecosystems perspectives<br>Developmental theory<br>Constructionist theory | Understand the person-in-environment assessment system<br>Identify specific areas where clients need change, specific problems of families and strengths of families in dealing with problems, and identify environmental contexts that need intervention<br>Employ theory-specific interventions |
| *DSM-IV*<br>Clinical disorders<br>Personality disorders and mental retardation<br>Psychosocial and environmental problems<br>Global assessment of functioning | Psychiatric theories<br>Ecosystems perspectives | Perform differential diagnosis to identify and understand the severity of mental disorders in family members<br>Recognize the limitations of formal assessment systems (in particular DSM-IV)<br>Recognize the impact of mental disorders on family functioning and health<br>Recognize the social context of disorder development and maintenance<br>Recognize the developmental progression of DSM-IV diagnostic conditions<br>Differentiate the need for individual and family interventions for DSM-IV diagnostic conditions<br>Ensure ethical decision making and oversee the diagnostic process<br>Practice addressing the question of "diagnostic fit"; suggested strategies for intervention and ethical decision making in diagnosis |
| *Resiliency Model of Family Stress*<br>Utilization of resistance resources by a family<br>Family's appraisal of a stressor situation and family's coping patterns<br>Maintenance of family function while dealing with a stressor<br>Identification of family's problem-solving ability | Family stress theory | Identify pileup of family stressors and determine interventions to reduce pileup<br>Recognize family patterns of functioning and target interventions to fit family type<br>Assess individual and family resources and develop strategies to enhance resource levels<br>Gauge extrafamilial social support levels and facilitate enhanced support resources<br>Recognize family schema and perceptions of family stressors and focus intervention to accommodate family perspectives<br>Identify family problem-solving skill level and offer interventions to strengthen the family's problem-solving resources<br>Apply the McCubbin family resilience model to allow a comprehensive assessment of pileup, patterns of functioning, resources, perception, and problem solving and develop an action plan fitting interventions to areas needing strengths building |

TABLE 16.1 *(continued)*

| Problem Focuses and Opportunities | Practice Theories | Practice Intervention Skills |
|---|---|---|
| *McMaster Model of Family Functioning and Family Assessment Device* | Systems theory<br>Role theory | Assess a family on seven dimensions of family functioning using the family assessment device and clinician rating scale |
| Assessment and identification of healthy family functioning and difficulties in family functioning | Communication theory | Prioritize the diagnostic information into treatment goals and problem resolution targets<br>Develop effective strategies to enhance family problem solving, communication, structure, affective involvement, behavior control, and commitment to its members |
| Assessing families strengths, concerns, resources, and priorities | Ecological theory<br>Family systems theory | Use genograms, Olson scales, family mapping, family and family member scales and environmental analysis, reframing, and family sculpting |
| *Family Functioning Considerations* | Family interventions | Use person-to-person relationship, emotional neutrality, genograms, and detriangling |
| Increase family members' differentiation and improve interdependence of family's emotional climate and behaviors | Bowenian family theory<br>Family systems theory | |
| Change in family organization or structure and change in the context of family transaction patterns | Structural family theory | Join and accommodate the family, make structural diagnosis, restructure the family, join the family, do enactment, mark boundaries, escalate stress, assign tasks, use paradoxical injunction, reframing, and mimesis |
| Replace dysfunctional family and individual behavior with more adaptive ones | Behavioral family practice | Complete behavioral baselines and presenting ground rules, communication skills, training, contracting, decision-making skills, conflict-management skills, modeling, cognitive restructuring and token economy |
| Effectiveness and assessment of practice intervention | Practice evaluation theory | Assess family functioning, outcome results, single-system designs, utilization of evaluation to enhance practice |
| Build frameworks for family health social work practice intervention by examining various family problems and developing an individual student's family intervention style for family health social work practice | Structural theory<br>Communications theory<br>Social learning theory<br>Family systems theory<br>Strategic family theory | Apply culturally and ethically sensitive practice principles to a wide range of family issues<br>Recognize the developmental issues with different family problems (e.g., family violence, blended family)<br>Apply strengths-oriented assessment and interventions to a wide range of family systems |
| Understand, identify, and practice intervention strategies for different family types | | |
| *Specific Practice Skills* | Structural family theory | Utilize confirmation, attitude, and behavioral reversal and joining |
| Demands that organize the ways in which families interact | | |

| Problem Focuses and Opportunities | Practice Theories | Practice Intervention Skills |
|---|---|---|
| Communication processes operating within family relationships (internal and external family communication) | Family communications theory<br>Family systems theory | Identify meta- and double-bind communication, use of metaphor, analogy, and reflective listening |
| Repeated sequences of behavior and dysfunctional hierarchies within the family | Strategic family theory | Apply directives and homework tasks, relabeling empowerment, straightforward directives, and paradoxical directions |
| Analyzing problems as a result of disruptive family functioning | Social learning theory | Apply behavioral reversal, contingency contracting, reinforcement (positive and negative), and contracting |
| Ethical decision making in family health social work practice | Utilitarian theory<br>Communication theory<br>Deontological theory<br>Egalitarian/libertarian theory<br>Virtue ethics<br>The ethics of care | Use of Joseph's model of ethical decision making which includes framing ethical dilemmas, gathering background information on the ethical dilemma, identifying and prioritizing values and biases, exploring options, and justifying an ethical position |
| Impact of social policies on family health | Ecosystems theory<br>Constructionist theory | Conduct policy analysis, i.e., rational, incremental, and criteria-based analytical skills |
| Political and organizational processes that influence family health | Systems theory<br>Constructionist theory | Use critical consciousness on allocation, provision, financing, and delivery of policy in relation to family health and policy formulation |
| Institutionalizing social policy | Ecosystems theory | Use cause advocacy, lobbying, and building networks of support, position taking, networking with political advocacy groups |
| Social and economic justice, diversity, and populations at risk | Constructionist theory<br>Systems theory<br>Ecosystems perspectives<br>Rawlsian theory of distributive justice | Promote empowerment, sensitivity to diversity, response to internalized oppression<br>Apply analytic skills to identify alternative policies and other practice interventions for dealing with social injustice<br>Develop political skills to assess policies' feasibility, identify power resources, and develop and implement political strategy to address issues of social and economic justice with populations at risk<br>Use interactional skills to make contacts, develop networks, build personal relationships, and identify influential networks<br>Use value-clarifications skills to consider the morality of certain policy proposals and strategies to obtain support for them |

TABLE 16.1 *(continued)*

| Problem Focuses and Opportunities | Practice Theories | Practice Intervention Skills |
|---|---|---|
| Focusing ethnic-sensitive practice on the values, identity, and cultural practices related to the family's ethnic group membership | Systems theory<br>Cognitive, affective, and behavioral theory<br>Constructivist theory<br>Role theory<br>Community theory<br>Organization theory | Engage in a culturally appropriate manner<br>Assess client in terms of problem and client's cultural and community perspective |
| Enhance emotional appreciation of ethnic-based dispositions and fears | Community theory<br>Organization theory | Use situational attending; contracting; ongoing reassessment of problem and partializing the problem<br>Apply advocacy role<br>Apply broker role |
| Adaption and modification of traditional strategies to accommodate the dual perspective of ethnic groups | | |

*Source:* Adapted from School of Social Work, Southwest Missouri State University (1998). *MSW Program Site Visit Response.* Springfield, MO: Author.

Assessment skills include appropriate use of DSM-IV, PIE (person-in-environment), and various family scales to create a diagnostic picture of individual, social, and family functioning; incorporation of empirical practice principles into service outcome assessment; and assessment of family policy effectiveness. Examples of such family scales include the McMaster Family Assessment Device (FAD) (Epstein, Baldwin, and Bishop, 1983), the Index of Family Relations (IFR) (Hudson, 1990), the Family Risk Scales (Magura, Moses, and Jones, 1987), the Family Adaptability and Cohesion Scales (FACES III) (Olsen, 1986), genogram, and ecomap.

Generalists' orientation to multilevels and multimethods practice provides the base for the family health social work practitioners. Certainly, wellness enhancement is not always best achieved within the walls of an interviewing room or within one family system. Policy intervention to produce more family-friendly policies or the development of additional resources within the community are just as powerful as effective therapy within a family unit.

## REFERENCES

Epstein, N., Baldwin, L., and Bishop, D. (1983). The McMaster Family Assessment Device. *Journal of Marital and Family Therapy, 9*, 171-180.

Hudson, W. W. (1990). *The WALMYR Assessment Scales Scoring Manual*, Temple, AZ: WALMYR Publishing.

Magura, S., Moses, B. S., and Jones, M. A. (1987). *Assessing risk and measuring change in families: The Family Risk Scales*. Washington, DC: Child Welfare Leagues of America.

Olson, D. H. (1986). Circumplex Model VII: Validation studies and FACES III. *Family Process, 26*, 337-351.

Pardeck, J. T. and Yuen, F. K. O. (1997). A family health approach to social work practice. *Family Therapy, 24*(2), 115-128.

Pardeck, J. T. and Yuen, F. K. O. (Eds.) (1999). *Family health: A holistic approach to social work practice*. Westport, CT: Auburn House.

Pardeck, J. T., Yuen, F. K. O., Daley, J., and Hawkins, C. (1998). Social work assessment and intervention through family health practice. *Family Therapy, 1*(25), 25-39.

School of Social Work, Southwest Missouri State University (SMSU) (1996). *A working paper on family health*. Springfield, MO: Author.

School of Social Work, Southwest Missouri State University (SMSU) (1998). *MSW program site visit response*. Springfield, MO: Author.

# Chapter 17

# Conclusions

## John T. Pardeck

Family health social work practice represents a departure from the dominant practice models that have been used by the helping professions. Family health social work practice has its seminal roots in the pioneering work of Mary Richmond. Given this tradition of focusing on the family system, the family health practitioner is well grounded in a theoretical orientation unique to the field of social work. Keeping this point in mind, the following basic premises guide the family health approach to social work practice:

1. Family health social work practice is grounded in a biopsychosocial approach to assessment and intervention; it rejects the narrowness of the biomedical model as a practice approach.
2. Family health is based on a systems-ecological approach to practice because of the role that various systems play in the well-being of the family. These systems include the person, the community, and the larger social context, which includes the numerous social systems that impact family functioning.
3. Family health views the family as the most important system for promoting the growth and development of the person.
4. Family health social work practice requires close collaboration between social workers and other professionals. The complexity of problems facing families demands the help of many professionals; social workers must be able to work with these groups.

One critical issue concerning the theoretical grounding of family health social work practice is the rejection of the biomedical model by practitioners who use this emerging paradigm. A family health social work perspective fully integrates the biopsychosocial aspects of a presenting problem. The family is seen as a dynamic system that helps to maintain health, offers support to family members, affects health decisions, and attaches meaning to illness. The client is viewed as an entity that affects and is affected by the family system. Assessment and intervention from a family health perspective involve the biopsychosocial aspects of not only the individual but also the entire family system (Pardeck and Yuen, 2001). What is powerful about the family health perspective is that an extensive body of research supports the need to conduct assessment and intervention from a biopsychosocial orientation in order to enhance practice effectiveness (Pardeck and Yuen, 2001).

As mentioned in Chapter 1, family health social work practice is guided by sound premises based on social scientific research. Campbell's (1986) findings mentioned in Chapter 1 are summarized in the following:

1. The family's impact on physical health is primarily derived from social epidemiology data and views the family as a potential source of stress on social supports. Studies suggest family interaction may play a role in the development of diabetes and asthma in family members.
2. Marital status and support by the spouse are potent family factors affecting overall mortality and cardiovascular disease. Bereavement is correlated with an increased risk of death in widowers. Family support, particularly by the spouse, has a protective effect that is not specific to any disease process.
3. Family intervention, such as involving the spouse in the case of a hypertensive client, can have an impact, and has been shown to lower overall mortality. In hypertension, the impact of family involvement is primarily due to increased compliance with antihypertensive medications and diet.
4. No evidence exists to demonstrate that family characteristics are associated with any specific illnesses. Empirical support for the concept of "psychosomatic families" is limited. Whether some physical illnesses are more influenced by family processes than others is also unknown.
5. Poor diabetic control is associated with family conflict and disorganization. Most studies of diabetic families conclude that poor diabetic control is due to lack of compliance with in-

sulin and diet. Minuchin's experimental work suggest that family interactions may have a direct effective on metabolic control.
6. A significant correlation between family support and compliance with medical regimens has been reported in cross-sectional studies only. Involving family members in the treatment of obesity helps promote weight loss.
7. Systems theory is the dominant paradigm in research on families with mental health problems. Patterns of family interaction have been found to be associated with particular illnesses.
8. Parental communication deviance is indicative of schizophrenic families and precedes the onset of fully developed symptoms. Adoption studies have shown an interaction between genetic factors and the family environment in the development of schizophrenia.
9. Studies of expressed emotions in families of schizophrenics offer the best evidence that the family system has an impact on health. Family therapy can affect emotional overinvolvement by the family, prevent relapse of symptoms, and reduce the need for hospitalization.
10. Depressed clients are sensitive to criticism by their families, and frequent critical comments by relatives are associated with high relapse rates. Marital discord frequently accompanies depression.
11. The interactions in alcoholic families are variable and depend on whether the alcoholic is in an abstinent (dry), drinking (wet), or transitional phase of the illness. During the drinking phase, interactional behaviors change during periods of intoxication. Observation of intoxicated behavior serving as an adaptive function for the family system has not been studied empirically.
12. The families of heroin addicts are characterized by rigid social interactions that include a dominant and overinvolved mother, a distant and passive father, and a dependent and addicted son or daughter. Family therapy may be more effective than individual treatment of drug addiction.
13. No patterns of family interactions correlated with anorexia nervosa have been empirically demonstrated.

Research by Ell and Northen (1990), McDaniel, Hepworth, and Doherty (1992), and Thompson and Pardeck (2000) can be summarized as follows:

1. How families react to stress appears to play a role in both the physical and mental health of family members.
2. The family system appears to shape health practices and health service use. The shaping of attitudes and behavior of family members' health practices is largely a result of the socialization process. Health-related behaviors include diet, exercise, tobacco use, and alcohol use.
3. The family has a clear and convincing influence on the psychological health of family members in both the theoretical and empirical literature. Examples of the family's impact on psychological health include preliminary evidence suggesting that family loss may be etiologically implicated in the development of health problems. Family coping styles appear to play a role in the development and reinforcement of coping behaviors of family members. Numerous studies report a relationship between family functioning and individual well-being. Research also reports that positive social supports offered by the family enhance family members' general well-being and the ability to cope constructively with stress.
4. The research provides persuasive evidence that the family plays a significant role in a family member's recovery from serious and life-threatening illness. Positive family support also appears to help clients better adapt to serious illness and to adhere to prescribed medical regimes.

In conclusion, the theoretical and social scientific literature supporting family health practice means social work practitioners are guided by an emerging paradigm that is effective at the micro-, mezzo-, and macrolevels of practice. This book has attempted to translate the theory and research supporting family health practice into a series of chapters focusing on assessment and intervention strategies in the traditional practice concerns of the profession, ranging from working with children who have been maltreated to intervention with clients in the mental health system. Each chapter attempts to illustrate that social work practice can be effective when grounded in the family health perspective.

## REFERENCES

Campbell, T. L. (1986). The family's impact on health: A critical review and annotated bibliography. *Family Systems Medicine, 4,* 135-328.

Ell, K. and Northen, H. (1990). *Families and health care: Psychosocial practice.* New York: Adline de Gruyter.

McDaniel, S. H., Hepworth, J. H., and Doherty, W. J. (1992). *Medical family therapy: A biopsychosocial approach to families with health problems.* New York: Basic Books.

Pardeck, J. T. and Yuen, F. K. O. (2001). Family health: An emerging paradigm for social workers. *Journal of Health and Social Policy, 13*(3), 59-74.

Thompson, R. and Pardeck, J. T. (2000). An exploration of the themes and content on family health in the social work literature. *Early Child Development and Care, 161,* 15-31.

# Index

Page numbers followed by the letter "f" indicate figures; those followed by the letter "t" indicate tables.

Accountability, family health agency, 152
Adaptation model, alcohol abuse, 114t, 115-116, 125
Adaptedness, ecological approach, 11
Administration
 ABC case study, 158
 family health agency, 147-148
Advanced generalist
 distinctiveness of, 35-36, 37
 social work practice, 14, 15, 16t
Advocacy
 ABC case study, 157
 cancer survivor case study, 172
 critical concerns, 19, 27
 family health agency, 151-152
 FHSWP skills, 206
Affective dimension, assessment, 44
African Americans, spiritual practices, 135-136
Al-Anon, Schutkin family, 62, 63
Alateen, Schutkin family, 62, 63
Alcohol abuse, problem of, 113
Alcohol dependence
 child sexual abuse, 58-59, 62
 example case study, 51-53
 family health research, 4
 family recovery models, 114t, 114-123
 and FHSWP, 124-125
 simulated case study, 125-127
Alcoholics Anonymous, Schutkin family, 62, 63
Alfred, domestic violence, 68, 71-72, 73, 74-75
Alicia, chronic pain syndrome, 195-197

Amanda, bipolar case study, 81, 82-83, 84, 86, 87, 89
*American Journal of Orthopsychiatry,* family health articles, 6t
Americans with Disabilities Act (ADA)
 description of, 161-162
 disability criteria, 163-164
 Harris opinion poll, 164
 human rights perspective, 171-172
Annie
 background, 137-140
 religious diversity case study, 140-145
Asian Americans, spiritual practices, 136-137
Assertiveness, example case study, 52
Assessment
 ABC case study, 155-156
 biopsychosocial continuum, 8-9
 bipolar case, 81-85
 cancer survivor case study, 168-170
 case example, 51-52
 case studies content, 43
 child sexual abuse, 57-58
 domestic violence case, 70-73
 elder caregiver case, 106
 Family Education and Support Program, 186
 family health, 3, 4
 and FHSWP, 43-46, 211
 ICN case study, 92-96
 religious diversity case, 140
Association for the Betterment of Community (ABC)
 background, 153-155
 case study, 155-159
Asthma, family health research, 4
Atherosclerosis, and stress, 7

*219*

Battered Women's Analysis: Batter-Generated Risks, 69
"Beanpole" family, 102
Beck Depression Scale, domestic violence, 69
Behavior, evaluation technique, 49-50
Behavioral dimension, assessment, 44
Behavioral patterns, ICN case study, 94
Behavioral/cognitive model, family counseling, 48, 208t
Biomedical model
  family health, 6-9
  FHSWP rejection of, 213
  and pain management, 193
Biopsychosocial model
  FHSWP premise, 4, 213-214
  pain case #1, 195-197
  pain case #2, 197-198
  pain case #3, 198-199
  pain case #4, 199
  pain case #5, 200
Bipolar disorder, case study, 81-89
Board of directors
  ABC case study, 158
  family health agency, 152
*Board of Trustees of University of Alabama v. Garrett*, job discrimination, 161
Bowen, Murray, 110
Bowenian model, family counseling, 48, 208t
Brian, bipolar case study, 81, 82-83, 84, 86-87, 89
Brown/Lewis model, alcohol abuse, 114t, 121-122, 124, 125, 126f, 128
Buddhism
  cultural support, 133
  religious diversity study, 139
Bush, George, and ADA, 161

Cancer survivors
  background, 165-167
  case study, 168-173
Cardiovascular disease, family health research, 4
Caregiver hierarchy, older adults, 102-103
Caregiver role, burden of, 103

Case advocacy, cancer survivor case study, 172
Case studies
  ABC, 155-159
  bipolar disorder, 81-89
  cancer survivors, 168-173
  content description, 42-43
  domestic violence, 68-77
  example case, 51-53
  family system, 175-180
  ICN family, 91-100
  older adults, 104-111
  pain cases, 195-200
  religious diversity, 137-145
  simulated, 125-127
Catholic Church, and Latino community, 136
Causality
  ecological approach, 11
  systems approach, 11
Cause advocacy, cancer survivor case study, 172
Change, process variable, 48
Chemical dependency, family health research, 4
Child sexual abuse, case study, 57-63
*Child Welfare*, family health articles, 6t
Child Well-Being Scales, ICN case study, 99-100
Child-rearing issues, Family Education and Support Program, 186-187
Children
  bipolar case study, 82-83, 84-85, 86-87, 88
  domestic violence case, 70-71, 74-75
  Family Education and Support Program, 185-187, 188
  homeless population, 31
  nutrition programs, 29-30
Christianity
  cultural support, 133-134
  religious diversity study, 139
Chronic pain syndrome
  case #1, 195-197
  case #2, 197-198
  case #3, 198-199
  case #4, 199
  case #5, 200

## Index

Civil Rights Act (1964), and ADA, 162
*Clinical Measurement Package, The: A Field Manual,* 46
Coalition building, domestic violence case, 76
"Codependence," 113
Cognitive dimension, assessment, 44
Cognitive-behavioral therapy, elder caregiver study, 110
Collaboration, family health premise, 4
Communication
  elder caregiver study, 106, 107, 109
  ICN case study, 93
Communication/experiential approach
  elder caregiver study, 110
  FHSWP, 208t
Communication/Strategic model, family counseling, 48
Community, ICN case study, 95
Compliance, family health research, 4
Confidentiality, ethical issues, 26
Conflict, caregiver role, 103
Conflict management stage, emotional systems model, 114t, 120
Confrontation
  Family Education and Support Program, 189
  FHSWP skills, 205
Confrontation stage, "taking charge" model, 114t, 121
Coping
  ecological approach, 11, 21
  strategies, example case study, 51
Council on Social Work Education (CSWE), ethics code, 25
Critical consciousness, concept of, 134
Cultural awareness, diversity, 22-23
Cultural competence
  description of, 22-24
  religious diversity study, 141
Cultural diversity
  bipolar case study, 88, 89
  description of, 22, 23-24
  and spirituality, 134, 135
Cultural pluralism, diversity, 22, 23
Cultural sensitivity, diversity, 22, 23
Cultural transformation, family function, 10

Curtis model, alcohol abuse, 114t, 117-118, 125
Custody, domestic violence case, 73

Data collection
  assessment techniques, 45-46
  domestic violence case, 68-69, 73
  elder caregiver case, 111
Denial stage, adaptation model, 114t, 115
Depression
  caregiver role, 103
  domestic violence, 69
  DSM-IV, 44
  example case study, 52
Descartes, Rene, 7
Developmental assessment, intervention skills, 205
Developmental assistance, Family Education and Support Program, 188
Developmental model, alcohol abuse, 114t, 117-118, 125
Diabetes, family health research, 4
*Diagnostic and Statistical Manual of Mental Disorders* (DSM-IV)
  depression, 44
  and FHSWP, 207t
  PTSD, 69
Diagnostic impressions
  ABC case study, 155-156
  bipolar case study, 81-85
  cancer survivor case study, 168-170
  case studies content, 43
  child sexual abuse, 57-58
  domestic violence case, 70-73
  elder caregiver case, 106
  example case study, 51, 52
  religious diversity study, 140
Dietary Guidelines for Americans, 30
Differentiation stage, emotional systems model, 114t, 120
Disability, ADA criteria, 163-164
Disabled
  and ADA, 161, 162
  discrimination against, 172
  nutrition programs, 29, 30
  as risk group, 26

Discrimination
   cancer survivors, 166
   disabled persons, 162-163
   and social justice, 26, 27
Disengagement stage, emotional systems model, 114t, 119-120
Disparate impact, ADA defense, 168
Disparate treatment, ADA defense, 168
Diversity
   critical concerns, 19, 22-24, 26-27
   and family system, 175, 176-177
"Diversity talk," 23
*Doctor, The*, 194
Domestic abuse, victim similarities, 65
Domestic violence
   ABC, 154
   case study, 68-77
   homeless population, 31
   theoretical approaches, 65-66
Don, ICN case study, 91-92, 93-94, 95, 96, 97, 98
Drinking stage, recovery model, 114t, 121-122
Dualism, biomedical model, 7
Duration, behavioral evaluation, 49-50
Duty to warn, ethical issues, 26

Early phase, phase model, 114t, 118-119
Early recovery stage
   developmental model, 114t, 118
   recovery model, 114t, 122
Ecological approach
   assessment, 45
   description of, 11-12
   domestic violence interventions, 66
   and FHSWP, 4, 19, 20f, 21, 207t, 208t, 209t
   limitations of, 12
   service provision, 147
Ecomap
   diagramming, 72
   elder caregiver study, 111
Education, bipolar case study, 86
Elderly. *See also* Older adults
   Medicare program, 31-32
   nutrition programs, 29, 30
Emotional nurturance, family function, 10

Emotional systems model, alcohol abuse, 114t, 119-120, 125
Employment discrimination
   ADA, 161, 168
   cancer survivors, 165
Employment skills, domestic violence case, 75
Empowerment
   Family Education and Support Program, 188
   FHSWP skills, 205
English Conversation Club, religious diversity study, 139
Environmental dimension, assessment, 44, 45
Equal employment officer, cancer survivors, 166-167
Equal Employment Opportunity Commission (EEOC), cancer survivors, 167, 169
Ethics
   critical concerns, 19, 26
   social worker codes, 25
Ethnicity, homeless population, 31
Evaluation
   ABC case, 159
   bipolar case, 88-89
   cancer survivor case study, 173
   case study content, 43
   child sexual abuse, 62-63
   domestic violence case, 76-77
   elder caregiver case, 111
   example case study, 51, 53
   family system, 180
   ICN case study, 99-100
   intervention strategies, 49-50
   religious diversity study, 144-145
Experiential/Humanistic model, family counseling, 48
*Explorations in Counseling and Spirituality*, 134

Faith, definition of, 131
*Families in Society*, family health articles, 6t
Family
   and biomedical model, 7
   biopsychosocial continuum, 8-9
   bipolar case study, 85

Family *(continued)*
 caregiver support, 103
 changed structure of, 102
 classification model, 72
 definition of, 9
 ecological approach, 11-12, 21
 Family Education and Support Program, 186-187
 family health perspective, 9-10, 47
 family health premise, 4
 family health research, 4-6, 6t
 FHSWP, view of, 214
 FHSWP definition, 203
 FHSWP dimensions, 204
 FHSWP skills, 206, 207t-210t
 ICN assessment, 92-96
 social policies, 28-32, 175-180
 social reality, 12
 stress, 207t
Family Adaptability and Cohesion Scales (FACES), assessment, 211
Family Assessment Device, 46, 53
Family Assistance Plan (FAP), family policy, 178
Family caregiver, older adults, 102
Family counseling
 intervention skills, 47-48
 theories of, 48, 207t, 208t, 209t, 210t
Family court system, domestic violence case, 75
Family disorganization stage, adaptation model, 114t, 115
Family Education and Support Program, family health perspective, 185-189
Family health
 biomedical model, 6-9
 definition of, 3, 6, 123-124
 FHSWP definition, 205
 practitioner roles, 189-190
 research findings, 4-6, 123, 214-216
Family health agency
 administration, 147-148
 agency, case study, 155-159
 organizational principles, 148-149
 versus family service agency, 149-153

Family health social work practice (FHSWP)
 agency services, 147-148
 biopsychosocial continuum, 8f, 8-9
 critical concerns, 19
 distinctiveness of, 35, 36-37
 ecological approach, 4, 11-12, 19, 20f, 21
 ethics code, 25-26
 Family Education and Support Program, 185-186, 189
 future developments, 37-38, 127-128
 goals of, 19
 intervention strategies overview, 41-42
 interventions checklist, 33, 34f, 35
 key concepts, 203-206, 207t-210t, 211
 premises of, 3-4, 213
 research, 123, 214-216
 social constructionism, 12-13, 19, 20f, 21, 43
 as social work field, 3, 5-6
 specialized practice, 13, 14-15, 16t
 and spirituality, 131, 132
 systems theory, 10-11, 12, 19, 20f, 21, 207t-210t
Family recovery, alcohol abuse, 113
Family recovery models, alcohol abuse, 114t, 114-123, 125
Family Recovery Project, recovery model, 121
Family Risk Scales
 assessment, 211
 ICN case study, 99-100
Family separation stage, adaptation model, 114t, 116
Family service
 domestic violence case, 75
 ICN case study, 93-94, 97, 99-100
Family service agency, versus family health agency, 149-153
Family system
 case study, 175-180
 problems of, 175
Feedback, systems approach, 11, 21
Feelings, assessment, 44
First Steps, ICN case study, 98, 99
Food Stamp Program, description of, 29

Frequency, behavioral evaluation, 49-50
Function, FHSWP dimension, 204

Gays/lesbians, risk group, 26
General Assistance (GA), public assistance, 29
Generalist
  distinctiveness of, 35, 37
  social work, 13-14, 15, 16t
Generalized Contentment Scale, 45-46
Genogram
  domestic violence, 72
  elder caregiver study, 111
Getting started stage, "taking charge" model, 114t, 120-121
GI Bill, voucher system, 179
Government
  ADA, 161
  and family system, 175, 176
Group counseling, domestic violence case, 75
Group theories, family practice, 49

Habitat, ecological approach, 11, 12, 21
Harris, Betty, alcohol dependence case, 125, 126, 127
Harris, Fred, alcohol dependence case, 125, 127
Harris, Katherine, alcohol dependence case, 125, 127
Harris, Tom, alcohol dependence case, 125-127
Harris public opinion poll, ADA, 164
Health
  definition of, 10
  FHSWP definition, 204
Health care
  domestic violence case, 75
  social justice, 31-32
Home visits, assessment practice, 43
Homelessness, social justice, 30-31
*Hospital and Community Psychiatry,* family health articles, 6t
Housing
  domestic violence case, 76
  social welfare programs, 30

Housing project, term, 30
Hudson, Walter, 45-46
Hurt, William, 194
Hypertension, and stress, 7

Identity, process variable, 48
Illness
  family response, 5
  psychoneuroimmunology, 7
Immigrants
  life stress, 132-133
  nutrition programs, 29
Income assistance policy, family policy, 177, 178-179
Income maintenance programs, description of, 28-29
Independence, biopsychosocial model, 195
Index of Clinical Stress, ICN case study, 100
Index of Family Relations (IFR), assessment, 211
Index of Marital Satisfaction, Schutkin family, 63
Index of Self-Esteem, ICN case study, 100
Individualism, and family system, 175, 176
Infants, domestic violence, 70
Information processing, process variable, 48
Informed consent, ethical issues, 26
Intensive care nursery (ICN), case study, 91-100
Intergenerational family therapy, elder caregiver study, 110
International Association for the Study of Pain (IASP), 193
Interval, behavioral evaluation, 49-50
Intervention plan, example case study, 52
Intervention skills, FHSWP, 205-206, 207t-210t. *See also* Intervention strategies
Intervention strategies
  ABC case study, 156-158
  bipolar case study, 86-88
  cancer survivor case study, 171-172
  case study content, 43

Intervention strategies *(continued)*
    child sexual abuse, 59-62
    description of, 47-49
    domestic violence case, 74-76
    example case study, 51, 52-53
    Family Education and Support
        Program, 186, 187, 190
    ICN case study, 96-99
    older adult case, 107-110
    religious diversity case, 141-144
Interventions
    biopsychosocial continuum, 8-9
    practice checklist, 33, 34f, 35
    sample questions, 21-22
Interviews, assessment technique, 45
Intimacy stage, emotional systems
        model, 114t, 120, 125
Islam
    cultural support, 133
    religious diversity study, 139

Jack, domestic violence case, 66, 67, 68
Jackson model, alcohol abuse, 114t,
        115-116, 125
Jenny, bipolar case study, 81, 84-85,
        87, 89
Jim, chronic pain syndrome, 200
Journals, family health articles, 6, 6t
Judaism, cultural support, 133

Kevin, domestic violence case, 67, 68
Knowledge, and values, 24

Late phase, phase model, 114t, 119,
        125
Late recovery stage, developmental
        model, 114t, 118, 125
Latinos, spiritual practices, 136
Lauren, domestic violence case, 67, 70
Law enforcement, domestic violence
        case, 76
Legal conflict, ADA defense, 168
Life stress, ecological approach, 11, 12,
        21
Lithium, bipolar case study, 81, 82, 86,
        88

Macrointervention, child sexual abuse,
        60-61
Macroskills, description of, 47
Magnitude, behavioral evaluation,
        49-50
Maintenance/remission stage,
        developmental model, 114t,
        118
Major life activities, ADA
        classification, 163
Management
    ABC case study, 158
    family health agency, 147-148, 153
Manic episode, bipolar case study, 81,
        82
Manifestations
    ABC case study, 156
    bipolar case study, 85
    cancer survivor case study, 170-171
    case study content, 43
    child sexual abuse, 58-60, 61-62
    elder caregiver study, 107
    example case study, 51
    family system, 175-177
    ICN case study, 96, 99
    religious diversity study, 141
Marital status, family health research, 4
Marital strain, child sexual abuse,
        58-59, 62, 63
Marital stress, bipolar case study, 83,
        87-88
Martinez, Anita, elder caregiver study,
        105, 106
Martinez, Carmen, elder caregiver
        study, 104, 105-106, 107,
        108, 110
Martinez, Manuel, elder caregiver
        study, 104-105, 106, 107,
        108, 109, 110
Martinez, Maria, elder caregiver study,
        104-105, 106, 107, 108, 110
Martinez, Roberto, elder caregiver
        study, 105, 106
Martinez family, elder caregiver case
        study, 104-111
Mary, bipolar case study, 81-89
Mary Ann
    background, 165-167
    cancer survivor case study, 168-173

*McDonnell Douglas v. Green,* job discrimination, 169, 170
McMaster Family Assessment Device (FAD), assessment, 211
McMaster model, domestic violence, 72, 208t
Meals on Wheels, nutrition program, 29, 30
Medicaid
 description of, 178
 Family Education and Support Program, 188, 190
 health care program, 31
Medical care, case study, 91-100
Medicare
 description of, 178
 health care program, 31-32
Mental growth/development, family function, 10
Mental health
 ABC, 153-159
 case study, 81-89
 family health research, 4, 5, 6
Mental illness, homeless population, 31
Mezzolevel interventions
 description of, 47, 49
 religious diversity study, 142
Microskills, description of, 47
Middle phase, phase model, 114t, 119
Middle recovery stage, developmental model, 114t, 118
Milan/Systemic model, family counseling, 48
Mortality rates, family health research, 4
"Motivational crisis," 117
Ms. Freeman, religious diversity study, 138-139, 141-142
Multiculturalism, diversity, 22, 23-24

Narrative approach, elder caregiver study, 110
National Association of Social Workers (NASW)
 ethics code, 25
 service provision, 147
National Coalition for the Homeless, homeless population, 31
National health insurance, family policy, 177, 178
National Law Center on Homelessness and Poverty, homeless population, 30-31
Native Americans, spiritual practices, 135
Nature, FHSWP dimension, 204
Negotiation stage, emotional systems model, 114t, 120
Niche, ecological approach, 11, 12, 21
Nixon, Richard, FAP, 178
Nutrition programs, description of, 29-30

Old Age, Survivors, and Disability Insurance (OASDI), 28
Older adults
 caregiver case study, 104-111
 and caregiving, 102
 population growth, 101
Ongoing recovery stage, recovery model, 114t, 122, 125
Oppression, social justice, 26, 27
Outcome-based planning, family health agency, 152

Pain
 biomedical model, 193
 biopsychosocial model, 193-195
 case #1, 195-197
 case #2, 197-198
 case #3, 198-199
 case #4, 199
 case #5, 200
 definition of, 193
 description of, 194
*Parachute kid,* 137
Parent/child relationships, spirituality issues, 143-144
Parents As Teachers, ICN case study, 98, 99
*Patch Adams,* 194
Pentecostal Latino church, and Latino community, 136

Personal Responsibility and Work Opportunity Reconciliation Act (1996), 29
Person-in-environment perspective, 41, 43, 44, 207t, 211
Phase model, alcohol abuse, 114t, 118-119, 125
Physical care, family function, 10
Planning, family health agency, 152
Policies, family health agency, 147, 148
Policing phase, process model, 114t, 117
Political advocacy
  ABC case study, 157
  family health agency, 151-152
Positionality, characteristics of, 134-135
Postmodern model, family counseling, 48
Post-traumatic stress disorder (PTSD)
  and domestic violence, 69, 71
  domestic violence case, 73, 74
Prejudice, social justice, 26, 27
Pretreatment stage, developmental model, 114t, 117
Prevention, FHSWP skills, 205
Prima facie case, establishing, 169
Primary caregiver, older adults, 102
Problem source
  ABC case study, 156
  bipolar case study, 85
  cancer survivor case study, 170-171
  case study content, 43
  child sexual abuse, 59
  description of, 46-47
  domestic violence case, 73
  elder caregiver case, 107
  example case study, 51-52
  family system, 175-177
  ICN case, 96, 98-99
  religious diversity case, 141
Process model, alcohol abuse, 114t, 116-117
Process variables, family counseling theories, 48
Provision of Social Relations scale, ICN case study, 100
Pseudomaturity, child sexual abuse, 61-63

Psychobiological dimension, assessment, 44, 45
Psychodynamic model, family counseling, 48
Psychoneuroimmunology, 7
"Psychosomatic families," 4
Public assistance programs, description of, 29
Public services/accommodations, ADA, 161

Random phase, process model, 114t, 116-117
Rathus Assertiveness Schedule, example case study, 52
Readiness, FHSWP skills, 205
Realization phase, process model, 114t, 117
Recovery, alcohol abuse, 113
Recovery model, alcohol abuse, 114t, 121-122, 124, 125, 126f, 128
Recovery stage, adaptation model, 114t, 116, 125
Recrimination phase, process model, 114t, 117
Refugees
  ABC, 154-155
  life stress, 132-133
Rehabilitation Act (1973)
  and ADA, 162
  and EEOC, 169
Relatedness
  ecological approach, 11, 21
  ecological assumptions, 12
Religion
  definition of, 131-132
  ethnic support, 133-134, 143
  and spirituality, 132
Research/practice evaluation, critical concerns, 19, 32-33
Resiliency Model, family stress, 207t
Resource allocation, ABC case study, 157
Resource coordination, family health agency, 150
Resource linkage
  Family Education and Support Program, 188
  intervention skills, 205

Retaliation, ADA, 161
Richmond, Mary, 3, 26, 213
Risk factors, assessment of, 27
Risk groups, critical concerns, 19, 26-27
Rita, domestic violence, 66-77
Roger, domestic violence case, 68, 70-71, 73, 74
Role structure
  elder caregiver case, 107, 109, 110
  process variable, 48
Roosevelt, Theodore, 178
Rosenberg model, alcohol abuse, 114t, 116-117
Ruth, chronic pain syndrome, 199

Safety plan
  for domestic violence, 69
  domestic violence case, 73
Sarah, chronic pain syndrome, 197-198
Satir, Virginia, 110
Schlesinger/Horberg model, alcohol abuse, 114t, 120-121, 125
Schutkin, Celine, child sexual abuse, 57-58, 59, 61, 62, 63
Schutkin, Jeremy, child sexual abuse, 57-58
Schutkin, Paul, child sexual abuse, 57-58, 59, 62, 63
Schutkin, Rebecca, child sexual abuse, 57-58, 59-60, 61, 62-63
Schutkin family, child sexual abuse, 57-63
Section 504, Rehabilitation Act, 162
Self-determination, ethical issues, 26
Self-Report Family Instrument, 46
Sexual issues, spirituality issues, 144
Sharon, chronic pain syndrome, 198-199
Skills
  case study content, 43
  types of, 47, 49
*Social Casework*, family health articles, 6t
Social constructionism
  domestic violence interventions, 66
  elder caregiver case, 110
  and FHSWP, 12-13, 19, 20f, 21, 207t-210t
Social constructivist, assessment perspective, 43
Social environment, critical concerns, 19
Social insurance programs, description of, 28-29
Social isolation stage, adaptation model, 114t, 115
Social justice
  critical concerns, 19, 26-27
  definition of, 26
Social learning approaches
  Family Education and Support Program, 189
  FHSWP, 205, 208t
Social Security Act (1935), 28, 178
Social services, family policy, 177, 179
Social welfare, knowledge/skills acquisition, 24
Social work
  educational preparation, 35-37
  FHSWP, 3-4, 8-9
  generalist approach, 13-14, 15, 16t
  professional values, 25
*Social Work*, family health articles, 6t
Socialization, family function, 10
Special Supplemental Nutrition Program for Women, Infants, and Children (WIC). *See* WIC
Spiritual diagnosis, 131
Spirituality
  bipolar case study, 88
  case study, 137-145
  child-rearing issues, 187
  definition of, 131
  domestic violence case, 74
  family function, 10
  FHSWP, 131, 132
  ICN case study, 92, 95, 97
  principles/practices, 134-137
  and religion, 132
Spousal relationships, spirituality issues, 143
Stabilization stage
  adaptation model, 114t, 115-116
  developmental model, 114t, 117
Stacy, ICN case study, 91, 92, 93-94, 95, 97, 98
Steinglass model, alcohol abuse, 114t, 118-119, 125
Stereotype, social justice, 26, 27

Strategic planning, family health agency, 149-150
Strengthening stage, "taking charge" model, 114t, 121
Stress
    caregiver role, 103
    domestic violence case, 73
    family health research, 5
    ICN case study, 98
    and illness, 7
    modern environment, 41
Structural family therapy, elder caregiver study, 109-110
Structural model, family counseling, 48
Structure, FHSWP dimension, 204
Substance abuse
    family recovery, 114-115
    prevention, ABC, 154
Suffering, description of, 194, 195
Supplemental Security Income (SSI)
    description of, 179
    public assistance, 29
Support, intervention skills, 205
Support system, domestic violence case, 76
Supportive intervention, Family Education and Support Program, 189
SWOT analysis, ABC case study, 156-157
Systems theory
    description of, 10-11, 21
    domestic violence interventions, 65-66
    family health premise, 4
    FHSWP, 19, 20f, 21, 208t-210t
    limitations of, 12

"Taking charge" model, alcohol abuse, 114t, 120-121
"Talking therapies," 53
Taoism
    cultural support, 133
    religious diversity study, 139
Ted, bipolar case study, 81, 82, 83, 86, 87, 88, 89
Telecommunications, ADA, 161
Temporary Assistance to Needy Families (TANF)
    FHSWP, 47
    public assistance, 29

Therapeutic relationship, domestic violence case, 74
Theresa, ICN case study, 91-92, 93, 94, 95, 96-98
Thriving stage, "taking charge" model, 114t, 121, 125
Transactions, ecological assumptions, 12
Transition stage, recovery model, 114t, 122
Treadway model, alcohol abuse, 114t, 119-120, 125
Treatment, alcohol abuse, 113
Truman, Harry, 178

Undue hardship, ADA defense, 168
Unemployment compensation, social insurance program, 28
U.S. Conference of Mayors, homeless population, 31

Values
    assessment, 44
    critical concerns, 19, 24-25
    definition of, 24
Veterans, homeless population, 31
Vouchers, social service, 179

WIC (Special Supplemental Nutrition Program for Women, Infants, and Children)
    description of, 29-30
    Family Education and Support Program, 188, 190
    ICN case study, 98, 99
Williams, Robin, 194
Women
    family caregiver, 102
    as risk group, 26
Workers' Compensation, social insurance program, 28

Zung Self-Rating Depression Scale, example case study, 52

## SPECIAL 25%-OFF DISCOUNT!
### Order a copy of this book with this form or online at:
http://www.haworthpressinc.com/store/product.asp?sku=4687

# FAMILY HEALTH SOCIAL WORK PRACTICE
## A Knowledge and Skills Casebook

_____ in hardbound at $29.96 (regularly $39.95) (ISBN: 0-7890-0717-7)

_____ in softbound at $17.21 (regularly $22.95) (ISBN: 0-7890-1648-6)

Or order online and use Code HEC25 in the shopping cart.

COST OF BOOKS_____

OUTSIDE US/CANADA/
MEXICO: ADD 20%_____

POSTAGE & HANDLING_____
(US: $5.00 for first book & $2.00
for each additional book)
Outside US: $6.00 for first book
& $2.00 for each additional book)

SUBTOTAL_____

IN CANADA: ADD 7% GST_____

STATE TAX_____
(NY, OH & MN residents, please
add appropriate local sales tax)

FINAL TOTAL_____
(If paying in Canadian funds,
convert using the current
exchange rate, UNESCO
coupons welcome)

☐ **BILL ME LATER:** ($5 service charge will be added)
(Bill-me option is good on US/Canada/Mexico orders only;
not good to jobbers, wholesalers, or subscription agencies.)

☐ Check here if billing address is different from
shipping address and attach purchase order and
billing address information.

Signature_____

☐ **PAYMENT ENCLOSED:** $_____

☐ **PLEASE CHARGE TO MY CREDIT CARD.**
☐ Visa ☐ MasterCard ☐ AmEx ☐ Discover
☐ Diner's Club ☐ Eurocard ☐ JCB

Account #_____

Exp. Date_____

Signature_____

Prices in US dollars and subject to change without notice.

NAME_____
INSTITUTION_____
ADDRESS_____
CITY_____
STATE/ZIP_____
COUNTRY_____ COUNTY (NY residents only)_____
TEL_____ FAX_____
E-MAIL_____

May we use your e-mail address for confirmations and other types of information? ☐ Yes ☐ No
We appreciate receiving your e-mail address and fax number. Haworth would like to e-mail or fax special discount offers to you, as a preferred customer. **We will never share, rent, or exchange your e-mail address or fax number.** We regard such actions as an invasion of your privacy.

Order From Your Local Bookstore or Directly From
**The Haworth Press, Inc.**
10 Alice Street, Binghamton, New York 13904-1580 • USA
TELEPHONE: 1-800-HAWORTH (1-800-429-6784) / Outside US/Canada: (607) 722-5857
FAX: 1-800-895-0582 / Outside US/Canada: (607) 722-6362
E-mailto: getinfo@haworthpressinc.com
PLEASE PHOTOCOPY THIS FORM FOR YOUR PERSONAL USE.
http://www.HaworthPress.com                                             BOF02